eQUALITY

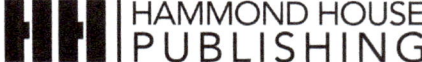

*© The Women's Exchange 2023
All rights reserved.*

No portion of this book may be reproduced, copied, distributed or adapted in any way, with the exception of certain activities permitted by applicable copyright laws, such as brief quotations in the context of a review or academic work.

Any similarities in this publication are purely coincidental.

For permission to publish, distribute or otherwise reproduce this work, please contact the authors Jill Wilson & Tracy Todd.

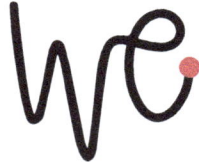

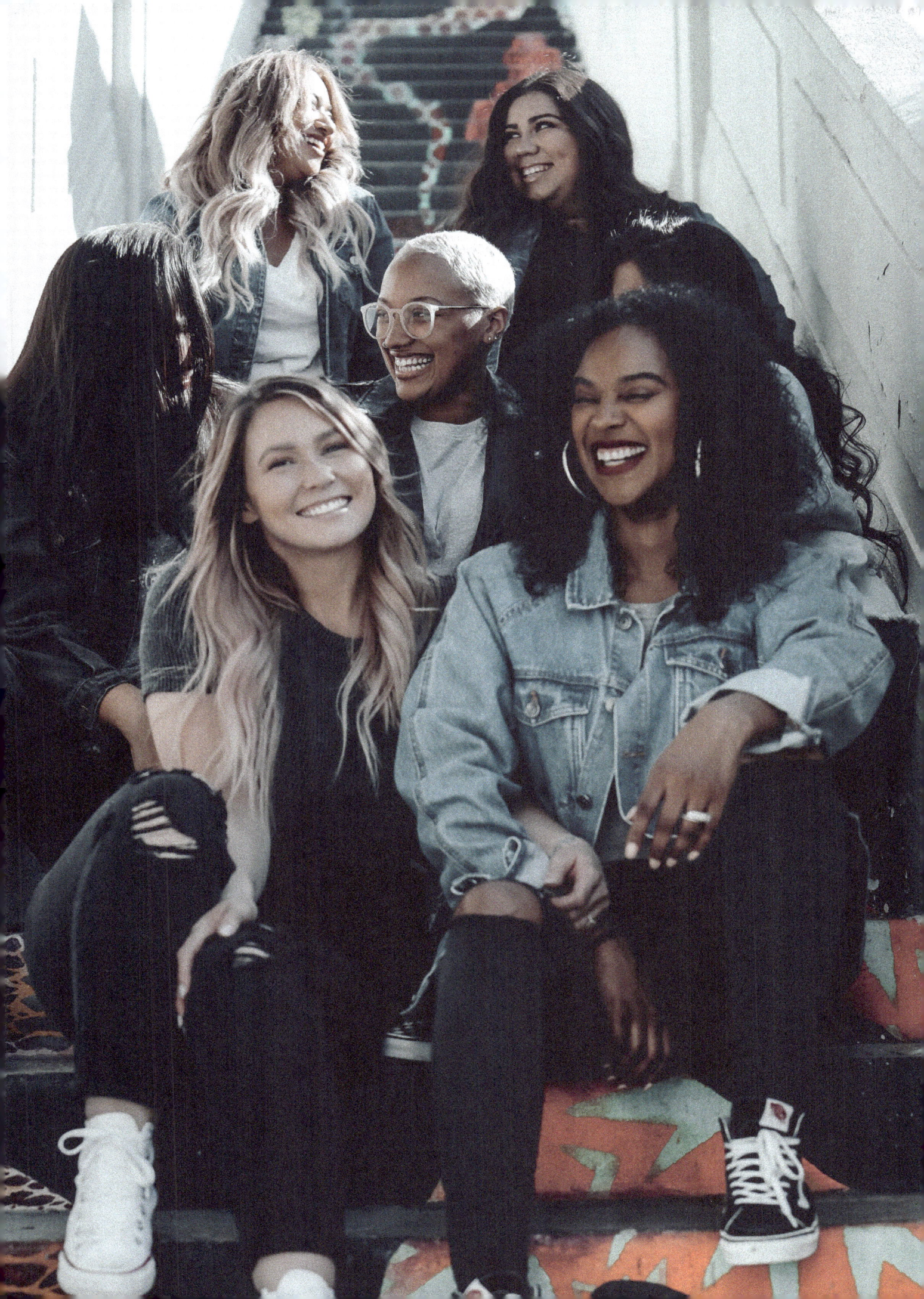

INTRO | ABOUT

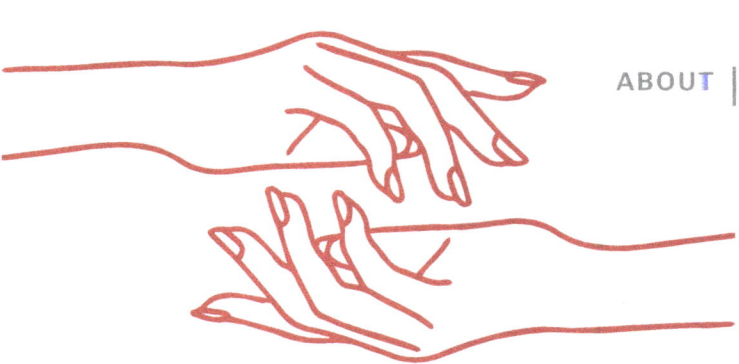

INTRO
ABOUT eQUALITY

So, let's crack on. eQUALITY has ten units; each unit has an online film which follows this ten-unit workbook. The really interesting and snazzy part of the course is the opportunity to interact and share with other women. This takes place on the forum, and is an integral part of the programme – we encourage you to fully participate in it. We also have the weekly live private Facebook sessions. If you cannot make them, they will be recorded. During these sessions, you will have the chance to share your learnings, ask questions and meet others taking the programme. Dates and times for the live sessions will be sent through to you.

Let's get this straight from the get-go. As with anything, the more you put into this programme, the greater the result you will achieve. Throughout you will be given instructions and asked to dig deep. Fully participating is your commitment to your transformation.

The purchase of this programme was the easy bit. However, financial investment alone is not enough to magically bring about the 'best you.' If only it was that easy!

We have been delivering this course for over seven years now and can confidently tell you that it works. Over 75% of all women experience life changing transitions. The only trick they used was they did all the activities and finished the course.

The eQuality Programme is all about YOU.

You ARE worth it. You will begin to retrain your brain to see yourself, your life and your goals in a new and different way. Everything you think, every way you think has been delivered to you by others, their expectations and how you have responded. Now's the time for you to begin re-thinking your thinking.

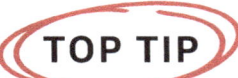

TOP TIP

Take your time. Don't rush each unit just because you can. Mull over your thoughts and feelings, let them find a resonating place to land. Absorb and reflect on what you do here, what you remember, realise and learn, then share your experiences on the forum. Do this throughout your time with us and practice the exercises away from your workbook and devices. The more you put into this course, the more you will achieve.

So, let's get on with this!

WARNING!

We can walk this road with you, but only you can make decisions for you and only you can make things happen. We are honoured you chose us and are looking forward to working with you.

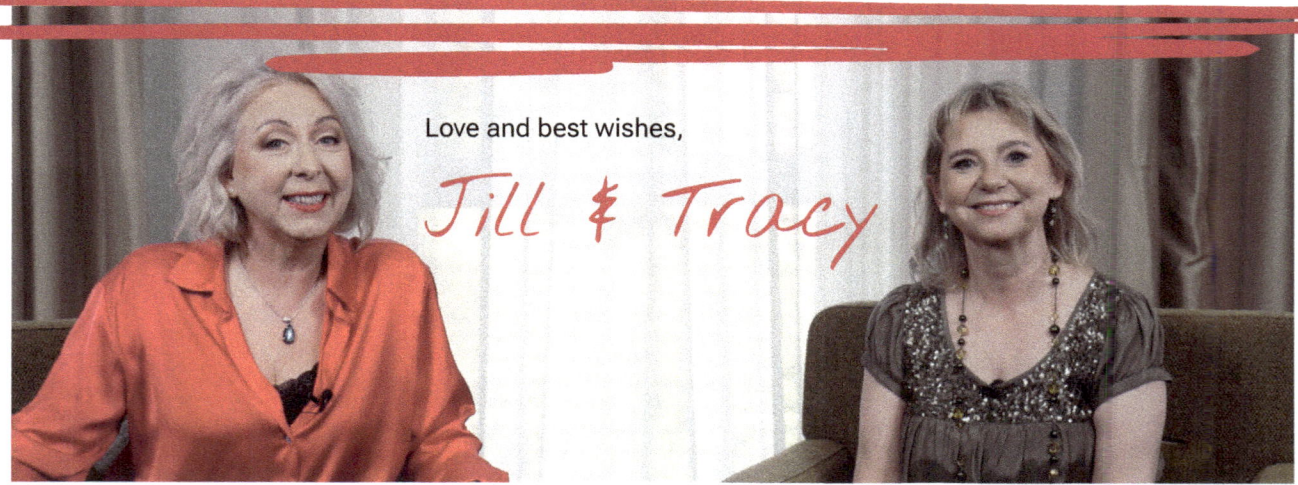

Love and best wishes,
Jill & Tracy

eQUALITY UNIT #01

'THINGS YOU LIKED THEN & NOW'

The why:
Let's Compare

This first unit focuses on looking back at ourselves when we were younger, comparing that with our present self and where we are now. How much of our younger self have we retained and how much has changed as we've grown older?

UNIT 01   'THINGS I LIKE'

ACTIVITY 01
LIKES WHEN YOU WERE YOUNG & NOW

What did you like to do when you were younger? Why did you like it? Do you still do any of the things you liked then, now? Have your likes changed since you were younger or are they the same?

Only go back as far as you are comfortable with. This may be childhood, teenage years or older. List the things you liked to do when you were younger and the things you still like to do now in the coloumns, below.

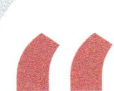
For in every adult there dwells the child that was and in every child there lies the adult that will be.

John Connolly,
The Book of Lost Things

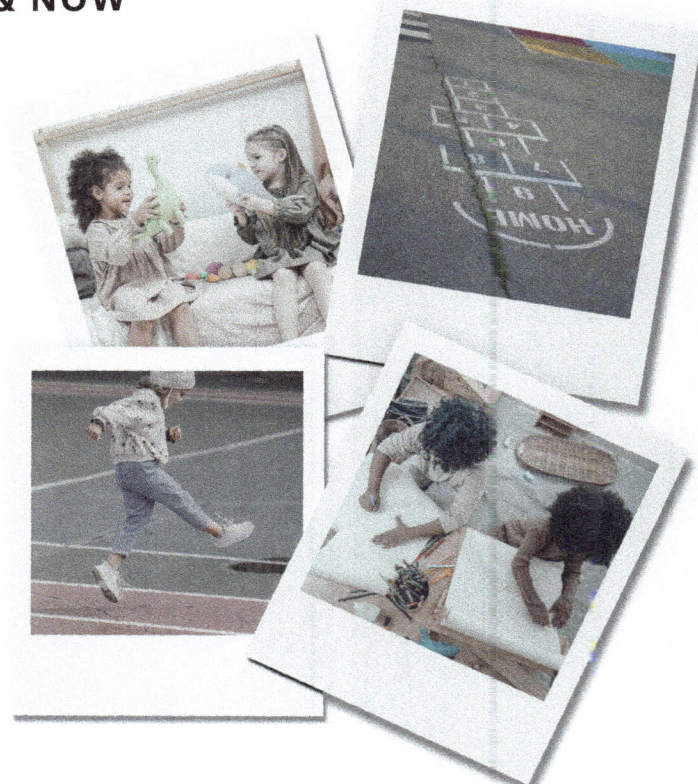

Younger

Now

UNIT 01 'THINGS I LIKE'

ACTIVITY 02
YOUR eQUALITY CHART

Your eQuality Chart is where you start your journey through this programme. You can download a blank chart, print it out or work on a computer. Once you have, complete the first two circles of your chart.

You may fill your chart with text, pictures, photos, objects. Be creative and be honest.

The outer circle (1) represents things you liked when you were younger.

The second circle (2) represents the things you like now.

In later units we will go on to explain the purpose of the other circles.

We don't often give ourselves time to think about who we were and who we wanted to be. Think about that now as you complete your chart.

Out of the dark, into the light

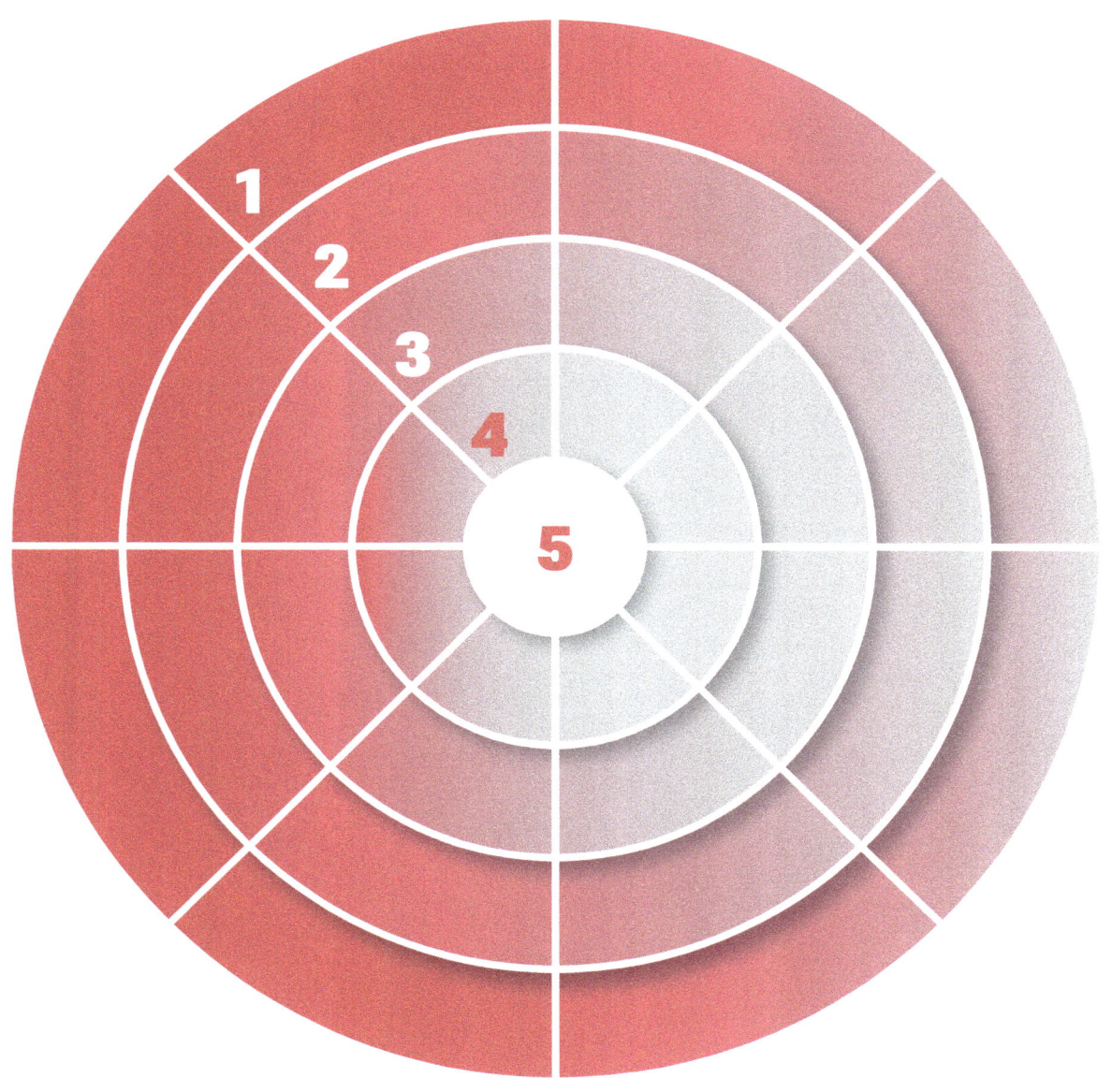

UNIT 01 | 'THINGS I LIKE'

EXAMPLE
eQUALITY CHART

This is Tracy's chart with the first two circles completed. The images were chosen from personal photos, images of books and videos.

Tracy's chart

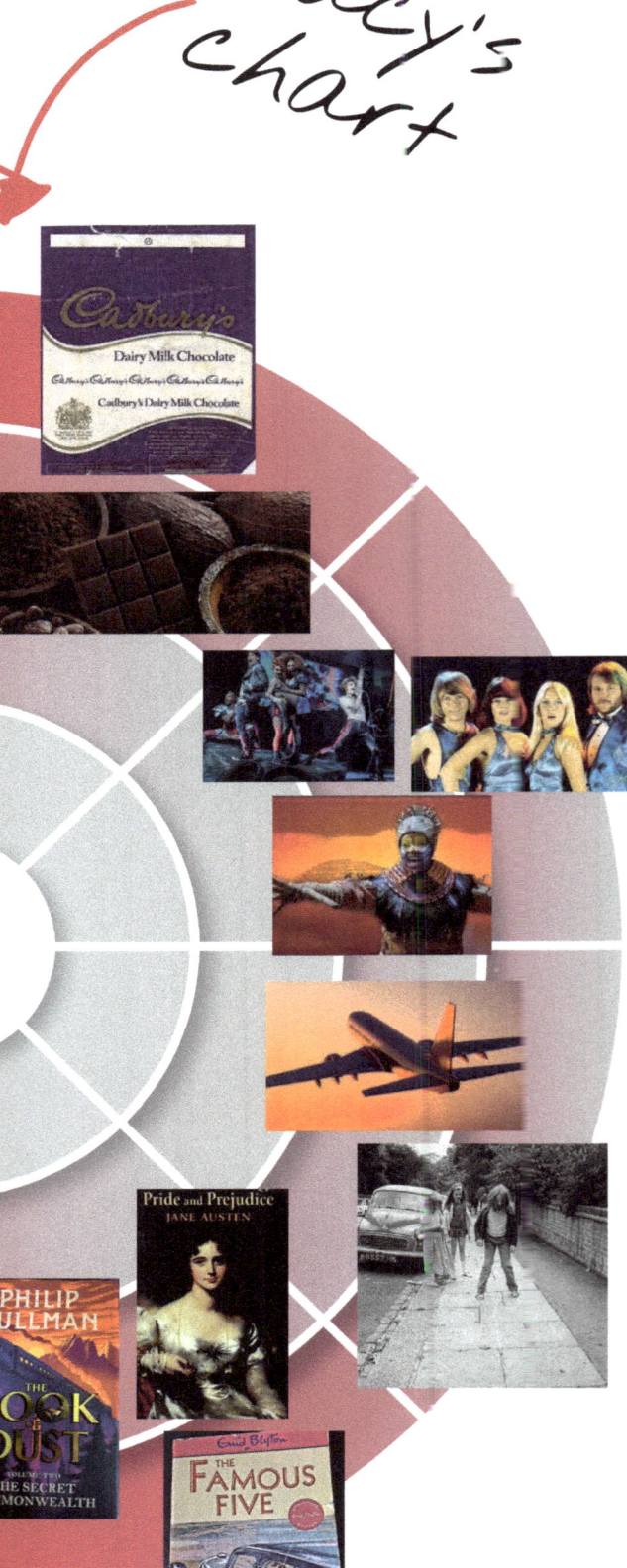

| UNIT 01 | 'THINGS I LIKE' |

REFLECTIONS
YOUR JOURNEY SO FAR

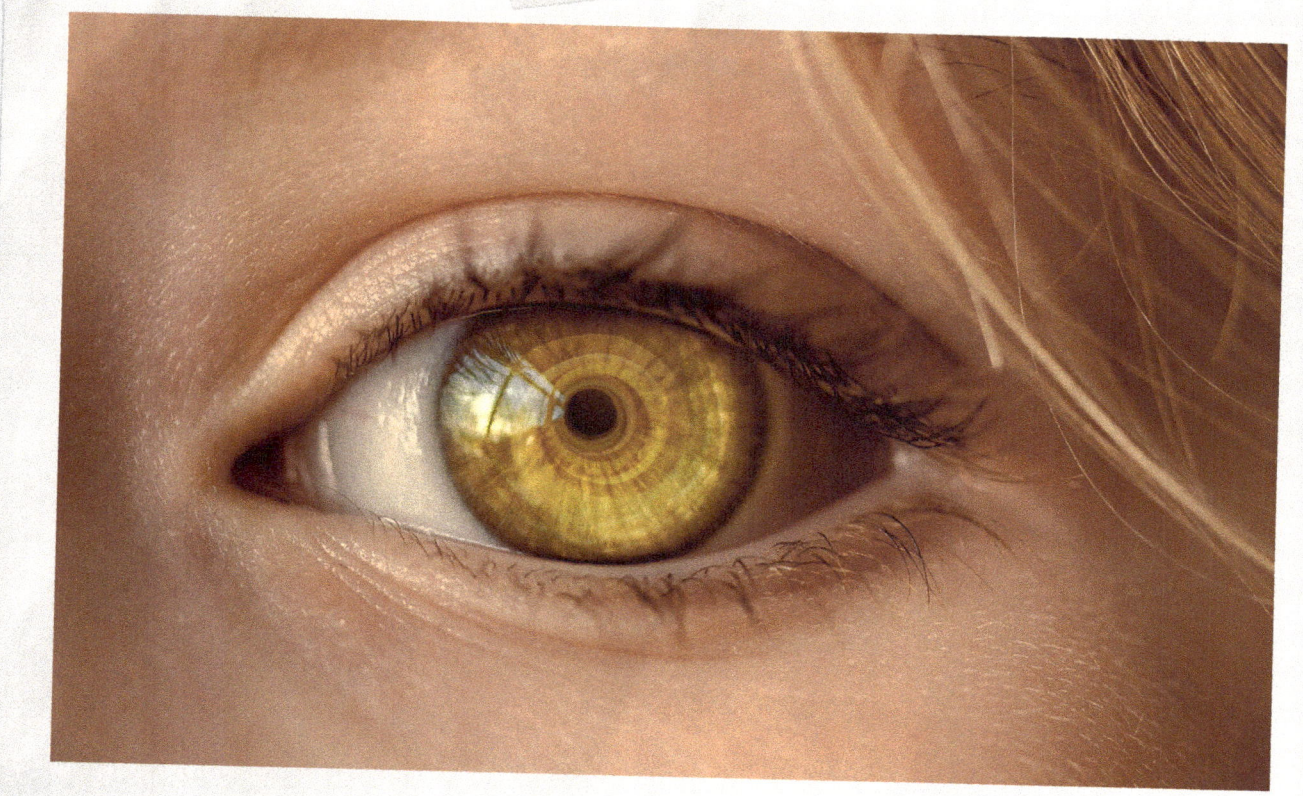

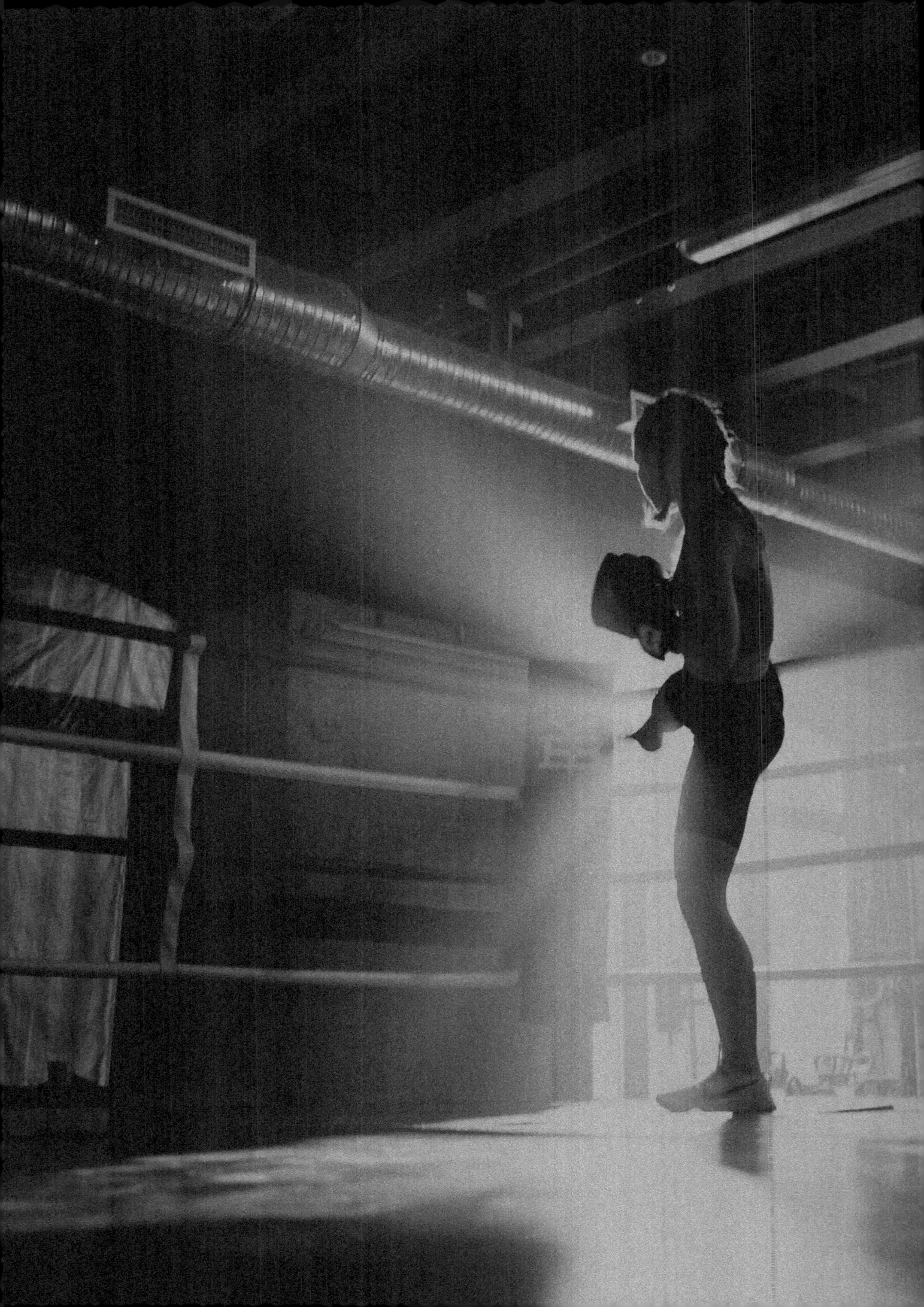

eQUALITY UNIT #02

'STRENGTHS'

The why:

It's time to think about our STRENGTHS.

Highlighting and talking about what we're good at may make us feel uncomfortable at first. We may not be used to it. But doing things that make us feel initially uncomfortable, such as talking about our strengths, will make us stronger.

| UNIT 02   'MY STRENGHTS' |

ACTIVITY 01
BRAIN TRAINING

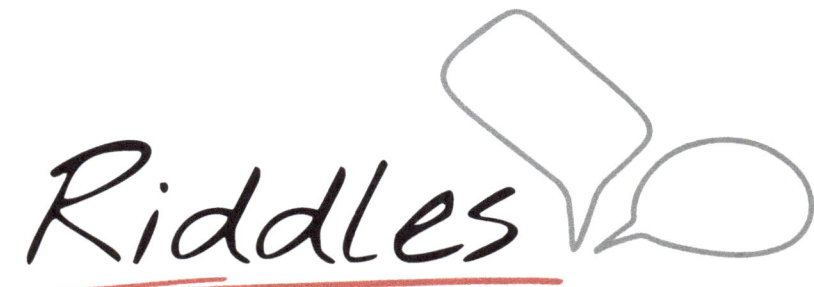

Riddles

01 What word begins with an 'e' and ends with an 'e', but only has one letter n it?

02 What ship has two mates but no captain?

03 Which five letter word becomes shorter when you add two letters to it?

04 What has a face and arms but no legs?

05 Three women were in a boat. It capsized, but only two got their hair wet. Why?

06 What has a neck but no face?

07 How many letters in the English Alphabet?

08 Why would a woman living in New York not be buried in Chicago?

09 What is so delicate that saying its name breaks it?

10 What gets wetter as it dries?

11 If everyone bought a white car, what would we have?

12 What begins with a 'T', ends with a 'T' and has 'T' in it?

THESE ARE GREAT TO SHARE WITH FAMILY & FRIENDS

UNIT 02   'MY STRENGTHS'

ACTIVITY 02
PERSONALITY QUIZ

> **This is a fun personality quiz.** Not to be taken too seriously. We want you to know if you are more like a Boudicca, a Marie Curie, a Kathrine Johnson or a Mother Theresa?

INSTRUCTIONS
In the space provided, identify the degree to which the following characteristics or behavior most accurately describes you at home or in relationships with your loved ones. When you've completed it, add up the number of words ticked in each column.

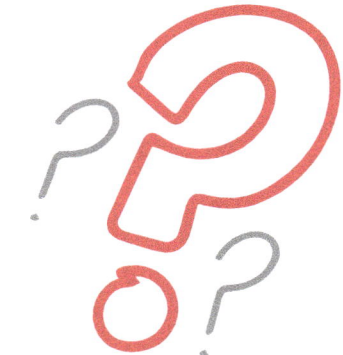

0 = NOT AT ALL | 1 = SOMEWHAT | 2 = MOSTLY | 3 = VERY MUCH

Coloumn 1	Coloumn 2	Coloumn 3	Coloumn 4
..... Likes Control	..... Enthusiastic	..... Sensitive	..... Consistent
..... Confident	..... Visionary	..... Calm	..... Reserved
..... Firm	..... Energetic	..... Non-demanding	..... Practical
..... Likes Challenge	..... Promoter	..... Enjoys Routine	..... Factual
..... Problem Solver	..... Socialises Easily	..... Relational	..... Perfectionist
..... Bold	..... Fun-loving	..... Adaptable	..... Inquisitive
..... Goal-driven	..... Spontaneous	..... Thoughtful	..... Persistent
..... Strong Willed	..... Likes New Ideas	..... Patient	..... Sensitive
..... Self-reliant	..... Optimistic	..... Good Listener	..... Accurate
..... Persistant	..... Takes Risks	..... Loyal	..... Controlled
..... Takes Charge	..... Motivator	..... Even-keeled	..... Predictable
..... Determined	..... Very Verbal	..... Gives In	..... Orderly
..... Enterprising	..... Friendly	..... Indecisive	..... Conscientious
..... Competitive	..... Popular	..... Dislikes Change	..... Discerning
..... Productive	..... Enjoys Variety	..... Dry Humour	..... Analytical
..... Purposeful	..... Group Orientated	..... Sympathetic	..... Precise
..... Adventerous	..... Initiator	..... Nurturing	..... Scheduled
..... Independent	..... Inspirational	..... Tolerant	..... Independent
..... Action Orientated	..... Likes Change	..... Peacemaker	..... Detailed
TOTAL SCORE	**TOTAL SCORE**	**TOTAL SCORE**	**TOTAL SCORE**

This was adapted from the online quiz at: www.smalley.cc

| UNIT 02 | | 'MY STRENGHTS' |

Your Score;

Simply plot your scores on the graph below, then connect the dots from one column to the next. Your strengths are the columns in which you scored the highest points.

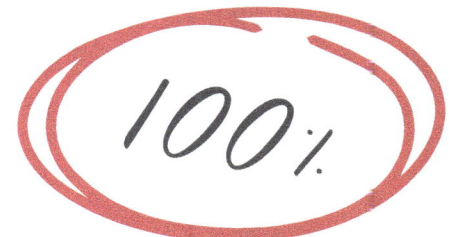

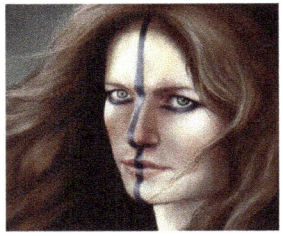
BOUDICCA

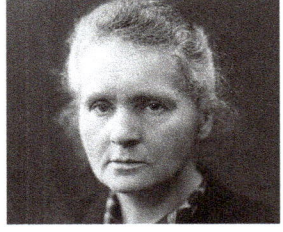
MARIE CURIE

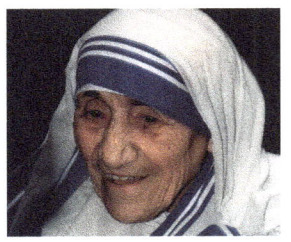
MOTHER THERESA

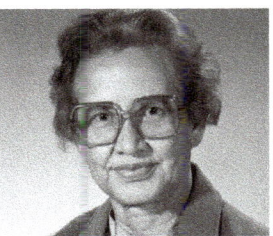
KATHERINE JOHNSON

60				
58				
56				
54				
52				
50				
48				
46				
44				
42				
40				
38				
36				
34				
32				
30				
28				
26				
24				
22				
20				
18				
16				
14				
12				
10				
08				
06				
04				
02				

UNIT 02 'MY STRENGTHS'

Sound like you?

Now read your interpretation. Does it sound like you? Are there any other strengths in the other columns that sound like you?

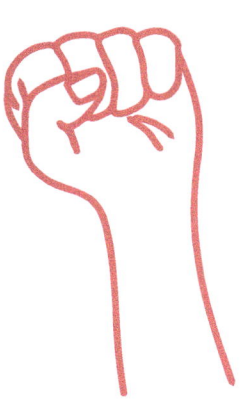

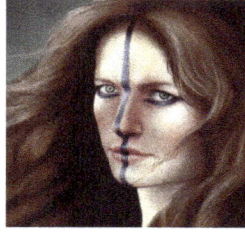
BOUDICCA
A warrior queen a queen of the Iceni tribe of Celtic Britons, who led an uprising against the conquering forces of the Roman Empire.

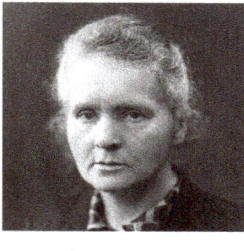
MARIE CURIE
First woman to win a Nobel Prize. Physicist & chemist who conducted pioneering research on radioactivity.

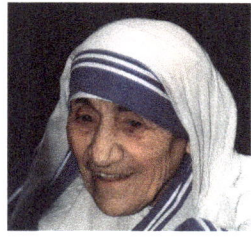
MOTHER THERESA
Catholic nun who dedicated her life to caring for the destitute.

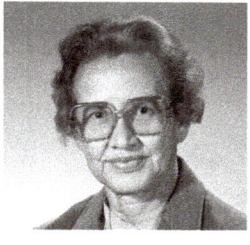
KATHERINE JOHNSON
Mathematician who worked at NASA. She solved equations by hand, as there were no computers, helping to get the first man on the moon.

	BOUDICCA	MARIE CURIE	MOTHER THERESA	KATHERINE JOHNSON
RELATIONAL STRENGTHS	Takes charge, problem solver, competitive, enjoys change, confrontational.	Optimistic, energetic, motivator, future orientated.	Warm & relational, loyal, enjoys routine, peacemaker, sensitive.	Accurate & precise, quality control, discerning, analytical.
STRENGTHS OUT OF BALANCE	Too direct or impatient, too busy, cold-blooded, impulsive, takes big risks, insensitive to others.	Unrealistic or daydreamer, impatient or over-bearing, manipulator or pushy, avoids details or lacks follow-through.	Attract the hurting, missed opportunities, stays in a rut, sacrifices own feelings for harmony, easily hurt or holds a grudge.	Over critical or strict, controlling, negative about new opportunities, lose overview.
COMMUNICATION STYLE	Direct or blunt, one-way. Weakness: not a good listener.	Can inspire others, optimistic or enthusiastic, one-way. Weakness: High energy can manipulate others.	Indirect, great listener. Weakness: Uses too many words or provides too many details.	Factual, great listener (tasks). Weakness: desire for detail, & precision can frustrate others.
RELATIONAL NEEDS	Personal attention & recognition for what they do, areas where they can take charge, opportunity to solve problems, freedom to change, challenging activities.	Approval, opportunity to verbalise, visibility, social recognition.	Emotional security, agreeable environment.	Quality, exact expectations.
RELATIONAL BALANCE	Add softness, become a great listener.	Be attentive to friend's needs, there is such a thing as too much optimism.	Learn to say "NO", establish emotional boundaries, learn to confront when own feelings are hurt.	Total support is not always possible. Thorough explanation isn't everything.

| UNIT 02 | 'MY STRENGHTS' |

ACTIVITY 03
KNOWING YOUR WEAKNESS IS A STRENGTH

Shereen is a single mum with two children, one aged 2, the other is 7. She has been working in a role she loves at a company that has supported her through pregnancy and divorce, but they don't seem eager to support her to progress in her career. She has been passed over three times now for promotion.

She is working in the world of Art, a world that she trained for, but lately she no longer feels fulfilled or appreciated. Her self-esteem is taking a hit and she is suffering from self-doubt.

There are plenty of senior roles in other sectors, but Shereen feels that if she moved sectors, she would lose connection with the world she loves and trained to be in.

Take a look at this scenario and identify Shereen's character strengths and skill set. Fill out the table below. Identify her weaknesses. Knowing our weaknesses is a strength. Can you say why?

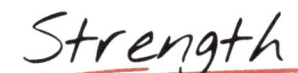

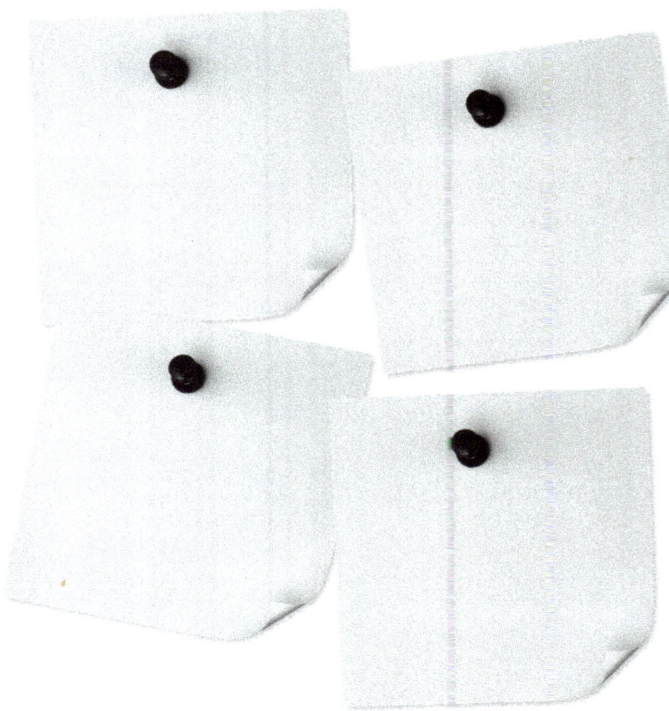

Is she doing the right thing, focusing on art only?

UNIT 02   'MY STRENGTHS'

ACTIVITY 04
STRENGTHS & WEAKNESSES

Think about your strengths. Jot down at least six character and skill strengths. Think about situations when you have used these strengths and remind yourself and others how strong you really are.

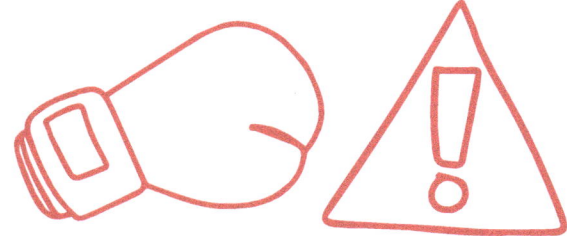

6 strengths

1.
2.
3.
4.
5.
6.

6 weaknesses

1.
2.
3.
4.
5.
6.

---

1. How are our strengths linked to our likes and passions?
2. Why is it good to be aware of weaknesses, but not focus on them?
3. How does all this affect our future?

UNIT 02 — 'MY STRENGHTS'

Quotes

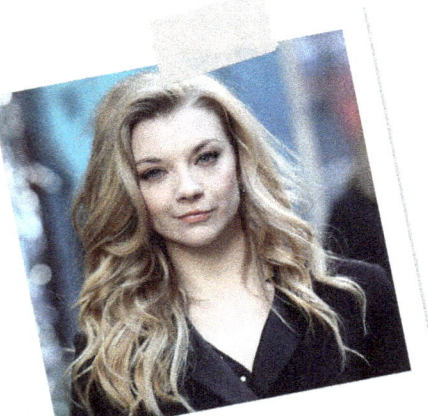

Q1. How does this quote relate specifically to learning and skills?

> For me, it's not necessarily interesting to play a strong, fearless woman. It's interesting to play a woman who is terrified and then overcomes that fear. It's about the journey. Courage is not the absence of fear, it's overcoming it.
>
> *Natalie Dormer*
> *Actress*

Q2. Are these statements true for me?
Q3. Are they talking about character or skill?

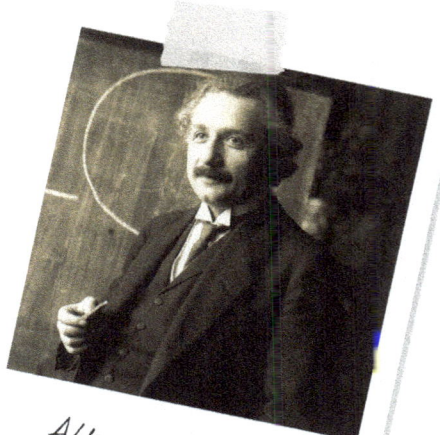
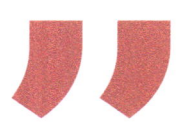

> Weakness of attitude becomes weakness of character.
>
> *Albert Einstein,*
> *Physicist & Philosopher*

18

ACTIVITY 05
CHARACTER STRENGTHS

> **Researchers have spent a lot of time** finding out which strengths of character are valued across cultures. They came up with a list of 24 character strengths. Tick which ones you think apply to you.

APPRECIATION	Noticing & appreciating beauty, excellence or skilled performance in all aspects of life	
BRAVERY	Not shrinking from threat, challenge or difficulty	
CAUTION	Not saying or doing things that might be regretted	
CREATIVITY	Thinking of new, productive ways to do things	
CURIOSITY	Taking an interest in experiences	
EMPATHY	Being aware of the motives & feelings of yourself & others	
ENTHUSIASM	Approaching life with excitement & energy	
FAIRNESS	Treating all people the same according to a sense of equality & justice	
FORGIVENESS	Forgiving those who have done wrong	
GRATITUDE	Being aware of & thankful for good things that happen	
HONESTY	Speaking the truth & being genuine	
HOPE/OPTIMISM	Expecting the best & working to achieve it	
HUMOUR	Liking to laugh & joke, bring smiles to other people	
KINDNESS	Doing favours & good deeds for others	
LEADERSHIP	Organising group activities & making sure they happen	
LOVE	Valuing close relationships with others	
LOVE OF LEARNING	Mastering new skills, topics & knowledge	
MODESTY	Letting your accomplishments speak for themselves	
OPEN-MINDEDNESS	Thinking things through & examining them from all sides	
PERSEVERANCE	Finishing what you start	
PERSPECTIVE	Being able to provide wise advice to others	
SELF-CONTROL	Controlling what you say & do	
SPIRITUALITY	Believing in the higher purpose & meaning of life	
TEAMWORK	Working well as a member of a group or team	

UNIT 02   'MY STRENGHTS'

Did you Know?

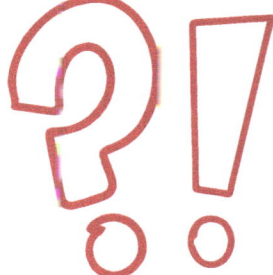

The most important character strengths for our wellbeing and happiness have been found to be:

- GRATITUDE
- OPTIMISM
- ENTHUSIASM
- CURIOSITY
- LOVE

Q1. What do these words mean to you?
Q2. Do you agree/disagree with any and why?

| UNIT 02 | 'MY STRENGTHS' |

REFLECTIONS
YOUR JOURNEY SO FAR

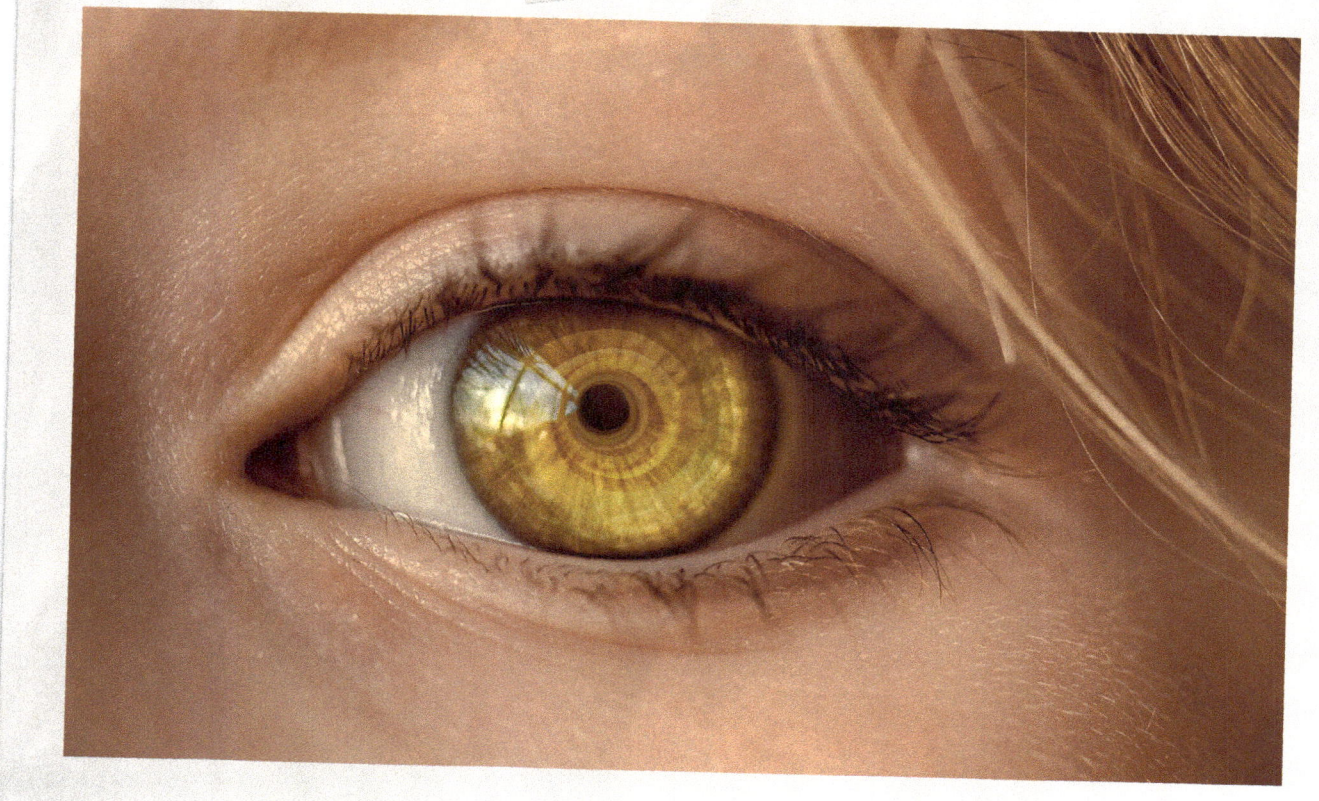

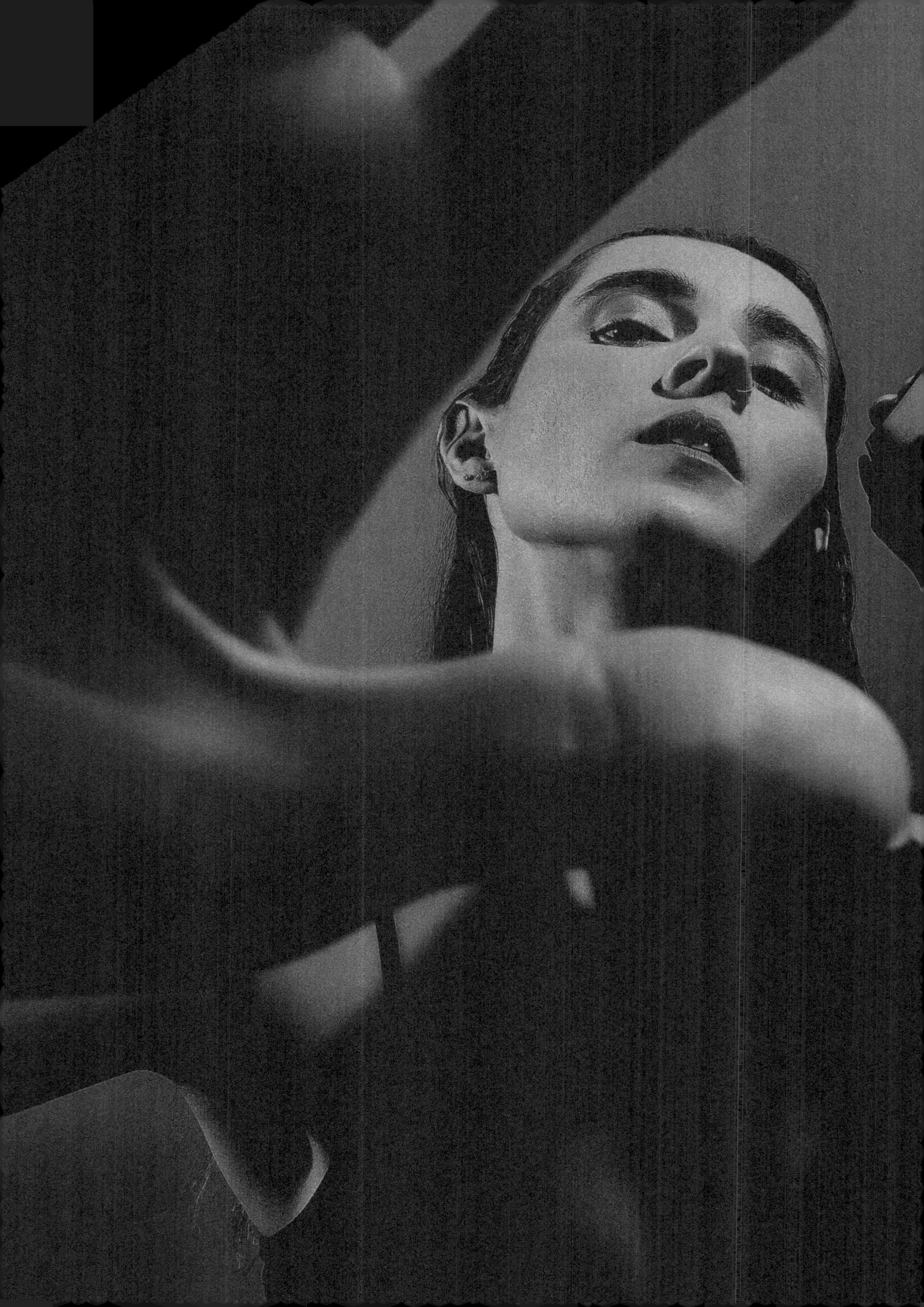

eQUALITY UNIT #03

'SELF-TALK'

The why:

Now it's time for some SELF TALK.

How do we talk to ourselves when we look in the mirror? Are we hyper-critical of ourselves, only noticing our faults? If that voice in our head is putting us down, that voice needs to change. To flip that negative, defeatist voice inside us is a Skill Strength, and it takes time. Changing our thinking and flipping those negative thoughts is a life-long practice. Empowerment starts now!

UNIT 03　　　　　　　　　　　　　　　　　　　　　'SELF-TALK'

ACTIVITY 01
WHAT DO YOU SEE?

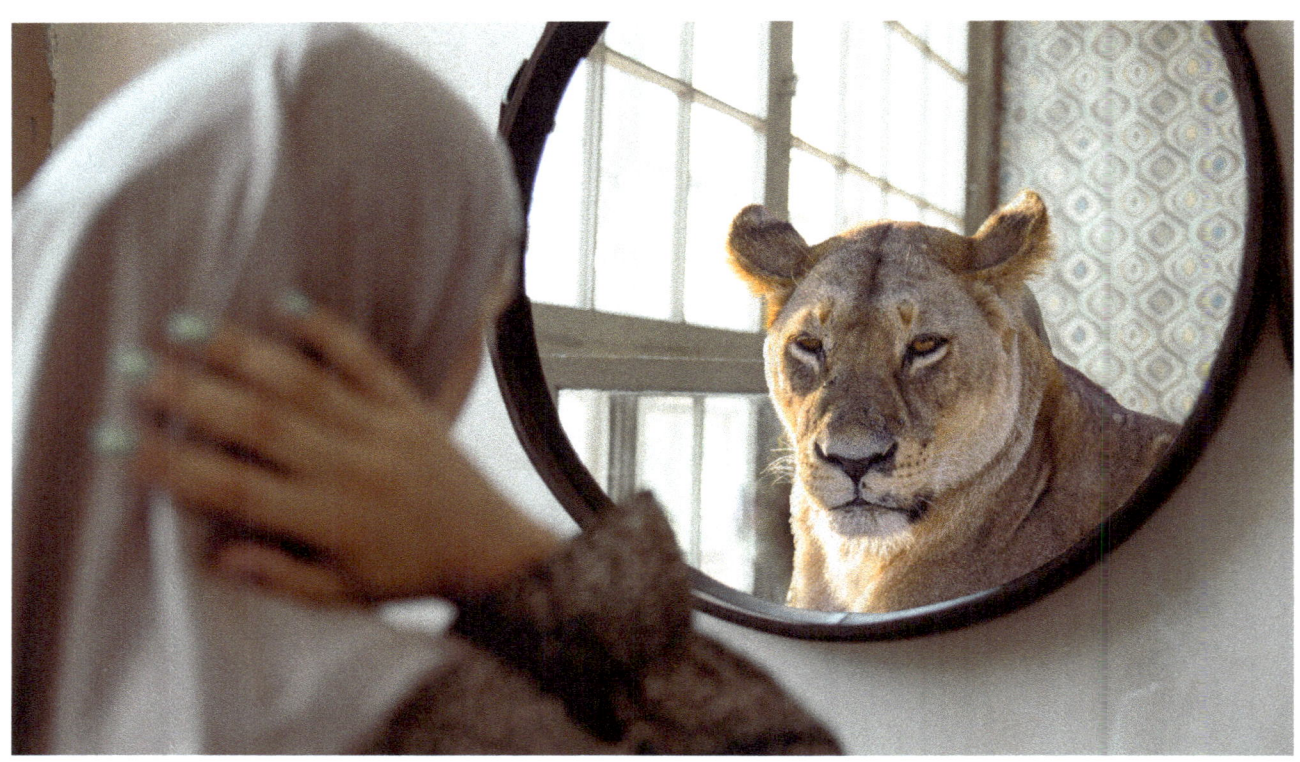

If I say, I can, or I say, I can't, I'm probably right.

Q1. What do these words mean to me?

Q2. Do I agree/disagree with any & why?

UNIT 03 'SELF-TALK'

ACTIVITY 02
CAN YOU RELATE?

Consider the two charts. Can you relate to them? Which would you prefer? Think about times when you have been content. Why were you content and how might you work towards it when you feel stressed?

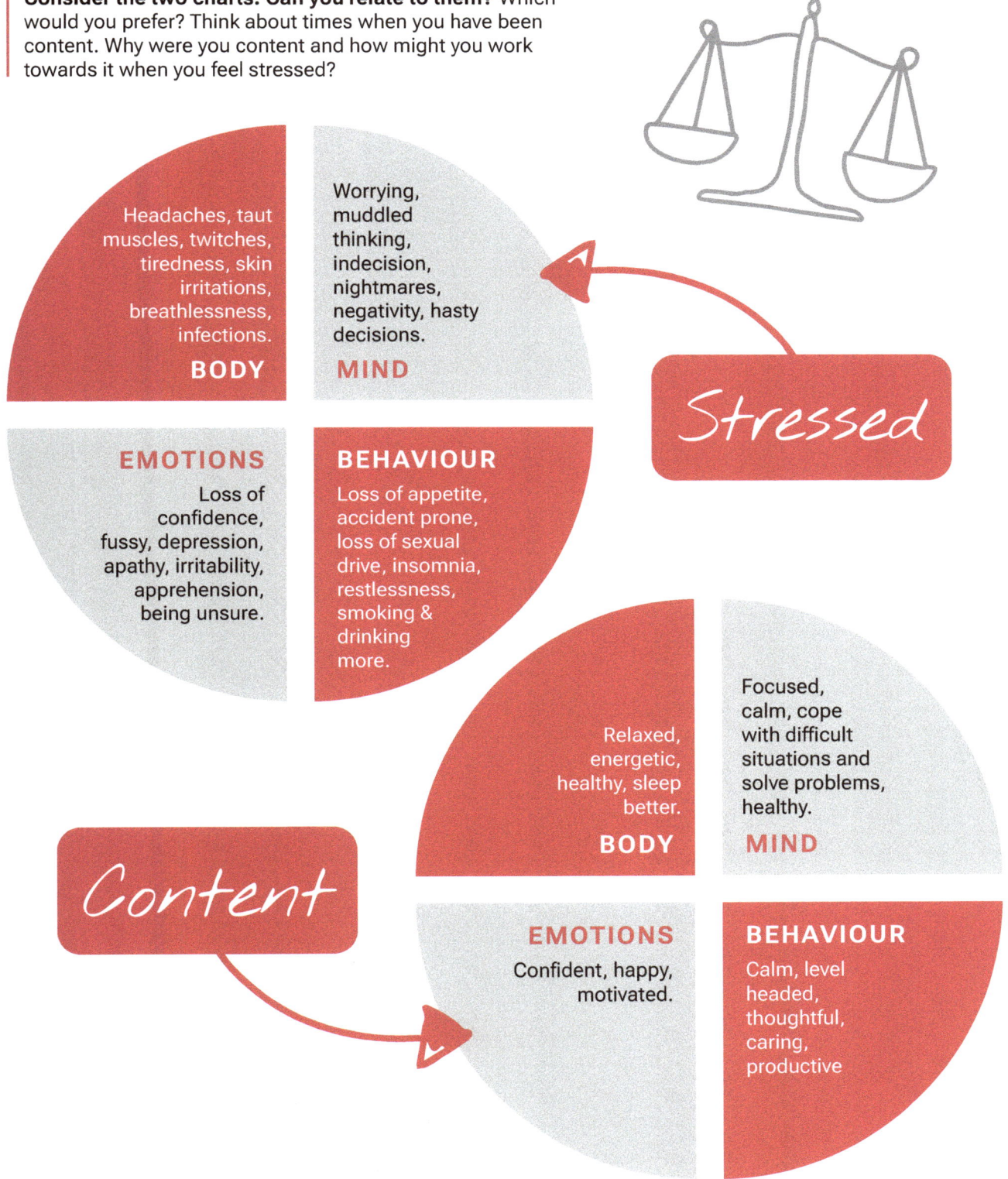

Stressed

BODY: Headaches, taut muscles, twitches, tiredness, skin irritations, breathlessness, infections.

MIND: Worrying, muddled thinking, indecision, nightmares, negativity, hasty decisions.

EMOTIONS: Loss of confidence, fussy, depression, apathy, irritability, apprehension, being unsure.

BEHAVIOUR: Loss of appetite, accident prone, loss of sexual drive, insomnia, restlessness, smoking & drinking more.

Content

BODY: Relaxed, energetic, healthy, sleep better.

MIND: Focused, calm, cope with difficult situations and solve problems, healthy.

EMOTIONS: Confident, happy, motivated.

BEHAVIOUR: Calm, level headed, thoughtful, caring, productive

If I say, I can, or I say, I can't, I'm probably right.

UNIT 03 'SELF-TALK'

ACTIVITY 03
FLIP YOUR NEGATIVE THOUGHTS

NEGATIVE THOUGHT	HOW DOES IT MAKE YOU FEEL?	FLIP IT	HOW DOES IT MAKE YOU FEEL?
I will never get a job. No one will choose me.	Bad about myself. Don't want to apply. Not worth it.	I will get a job. I will practice speaking about my strengths and experience. I will practice interviewing until I've nailed it.	More confident. Believe in myself.
I look awful.	First thing I say when I look in the mirror. Gets me down.	Wow... my skin looks good today. My hair is shiny.	Lifts my spirits. Makes me feel better about going out.

If I say, I can, or I say, I can't, I'm probably right.

Affirmations

Take a look below. Do you prefer any of the affirmations shown here? Choose one or two and practice saying them to yourself every day, or you can look for your own and use those.

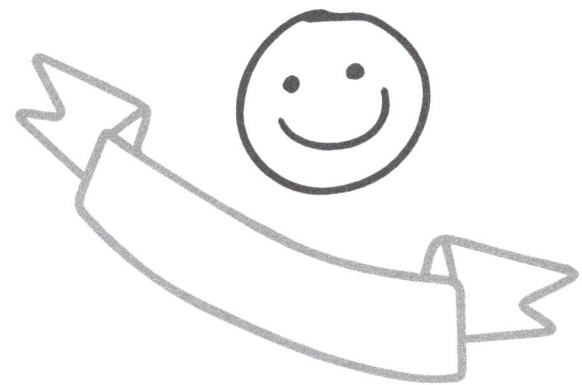

> **DON'T WORRY ABOUT FAILURES, WORRY ABOUT THE CHANCES YOU MISS WHEN YOU DON'T EVEN TRY.**
> *Jack Canfield*

> **YOUR MIND IS A POWERFUL THING. WHEN YOU FILL IT WITH POSITIVE THOUGHTS, YOUR LIFE WILL BEGIN TO CHANGE.**
> *Kamil Thomas*

> **ALL YOU CAN CHANGE IS YOURSELF, BUT SOMETIMES THAT CHANGES EVERYTHING.**
> *Gary W Goldstein*

> **EVERYTHING YOU'VE EVER WANTED IS ON THE OTHER SIDE OF FEAR.**
> *George Addair*

If I say, I can, or I say, I can't, I'm probably right.

UNIT 03 | 'SELF-TALK'

Affirmations

Take a look below. Do you prefer any of the affirmations shown here? Choose one or two and practice saying them to yourself every day, or you can look for your own and use those.

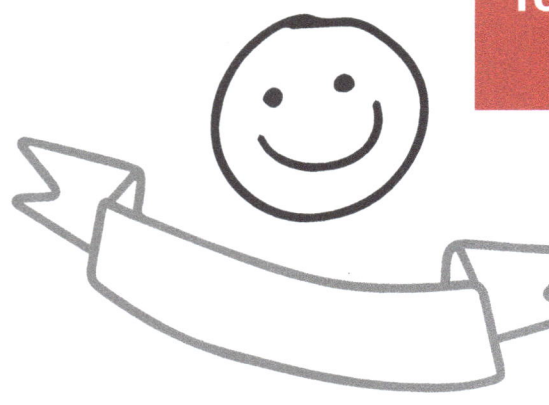

A SETBACK IS SIMPLY AN EXPERIENCE THAT WILL HELP ME GROW STRONGER.

I AM WORTHY OF LOVE. I AM WORTHY OF HEALING. I AM WORTHY OF PRIDE IN MY ACTIONS. I AM WORTHY OF GREATNESS.

I AM ALWAYS LEARNING AND GROWING.

I BELIEVE I CAN BE WHATEVER I WANT TO BE.

I FORGIVE MYSELF FOR ALL THE MISTAKES I HAVE MADE.

WHAT OTHERS THINK OF ME IS THEIR CHOICE, WHAT I THINK OF MYSELF IS MY CHOICE.

If I say, I can, or I say, I can't, I'm probably right.

UNIT 03 'SELF-TALK'

ACTIVITY 04
TOOT YOUR OWN HORN

Complete the statements. If you cannot put an answer to all, don't worry - simply complete what you can. Keep this handy. The next time you're feeling a bout of low self-esteem looming, take another look here and be reminded of your natural resources and personal power.

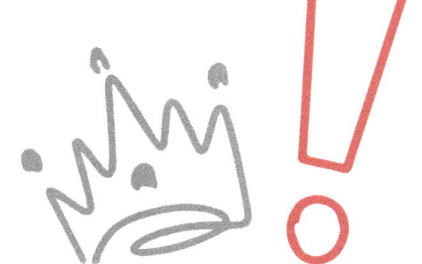

I like myself because:	
I'm an expert at:	
I feel good about:	
My friends would tell you I have great:	
My favourite place is:	
I'm loved by:	
People say I'm good at:	
I've been told I have pretty:	
I consider myself good at:	
What I enjoy most is:	
The person I admire the most is:	
I have a natural talent for:	
My goals for my future are:	
I know I will reach my goals because I am:	
People compliment me about:	
I feel good when I:	
I've been successful at:	
I laugh when I think about:	
The traits I admire myself for are:	
I feel peaceful when:	

If I say, I can, or I say, I can't, I'm probably right.

UNIT 03   'SELF-TALK'

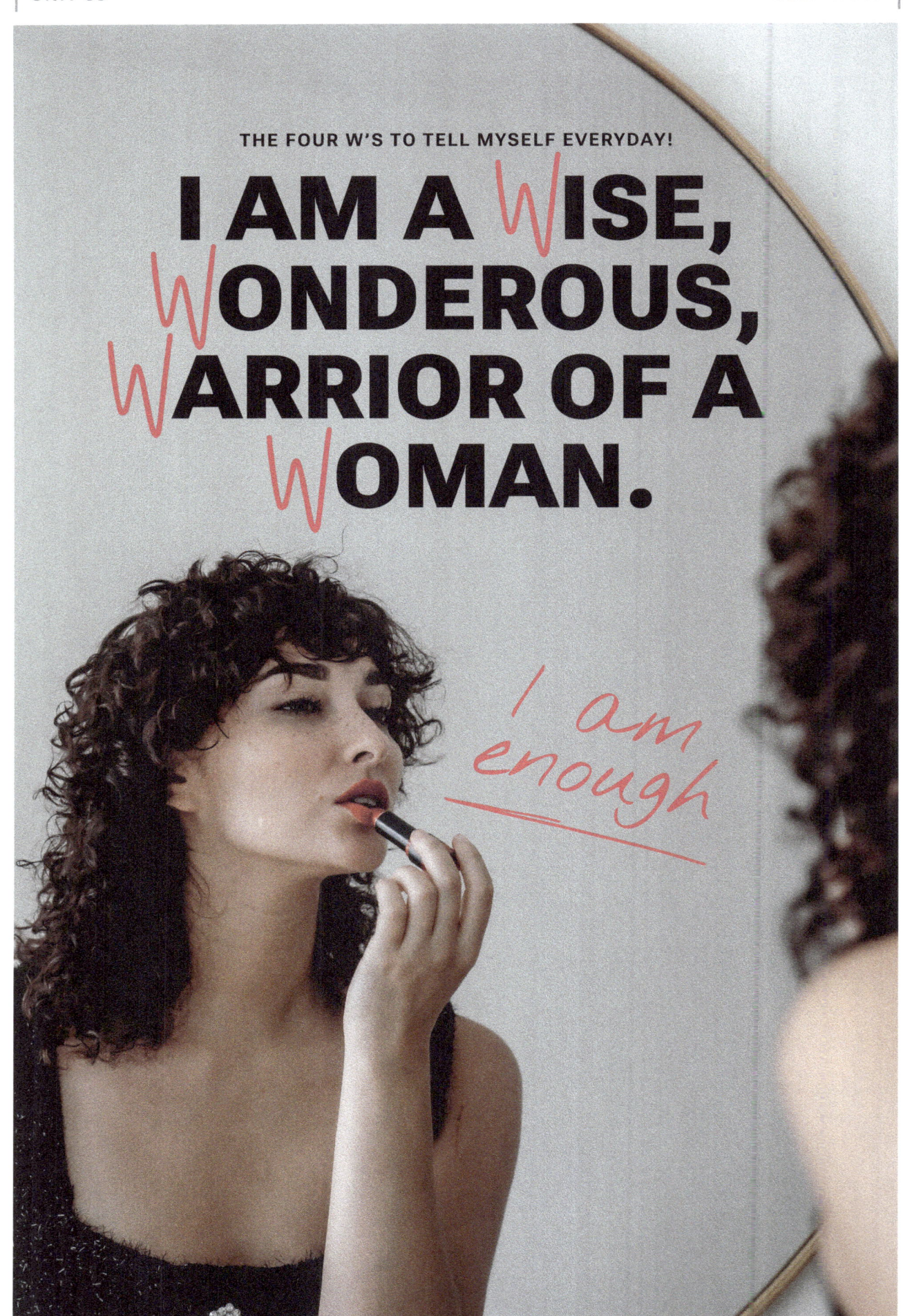

If I say, I can, or I say, I can't, I'm probably right.

UNIT 03   'SELF-TALK'

REFLECTIONS
YOUR JOURNEY SO FAR

If I say, I can, or I say, I can't, I'm probably right. What does this mean...

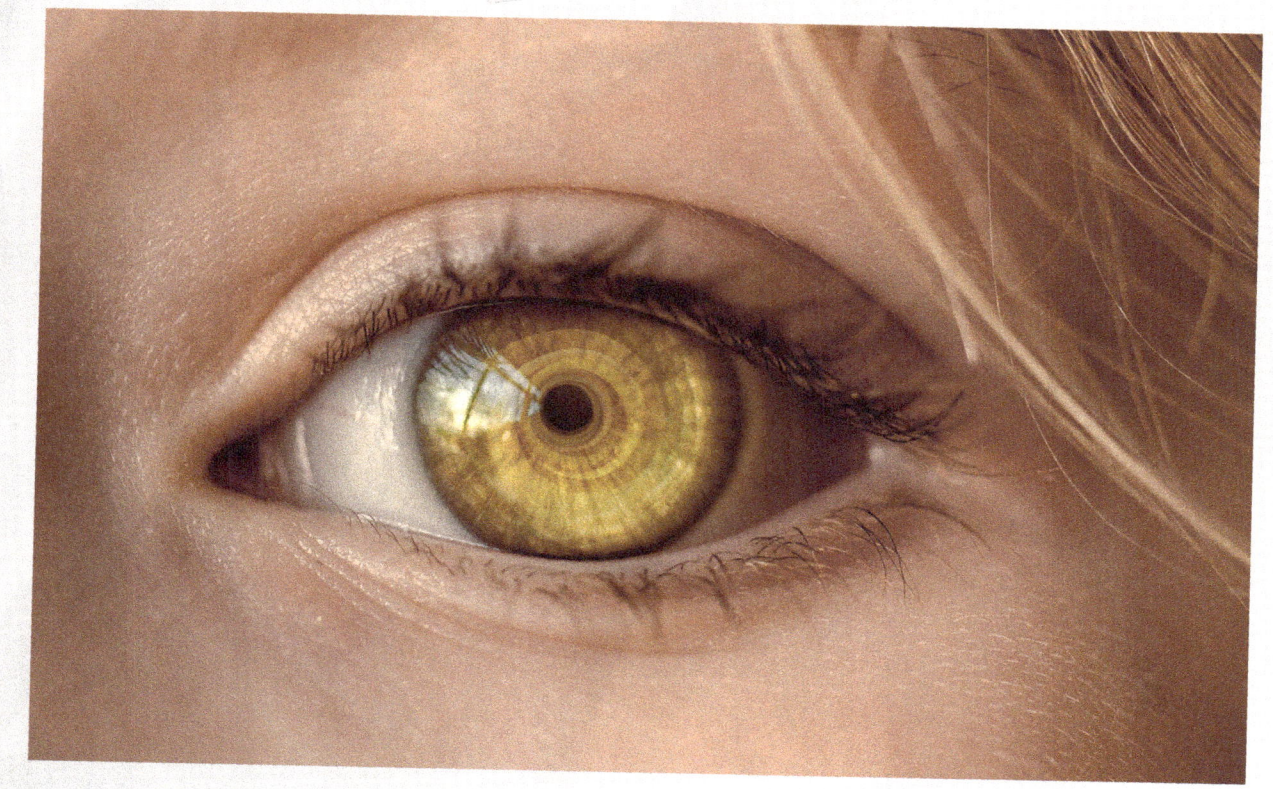

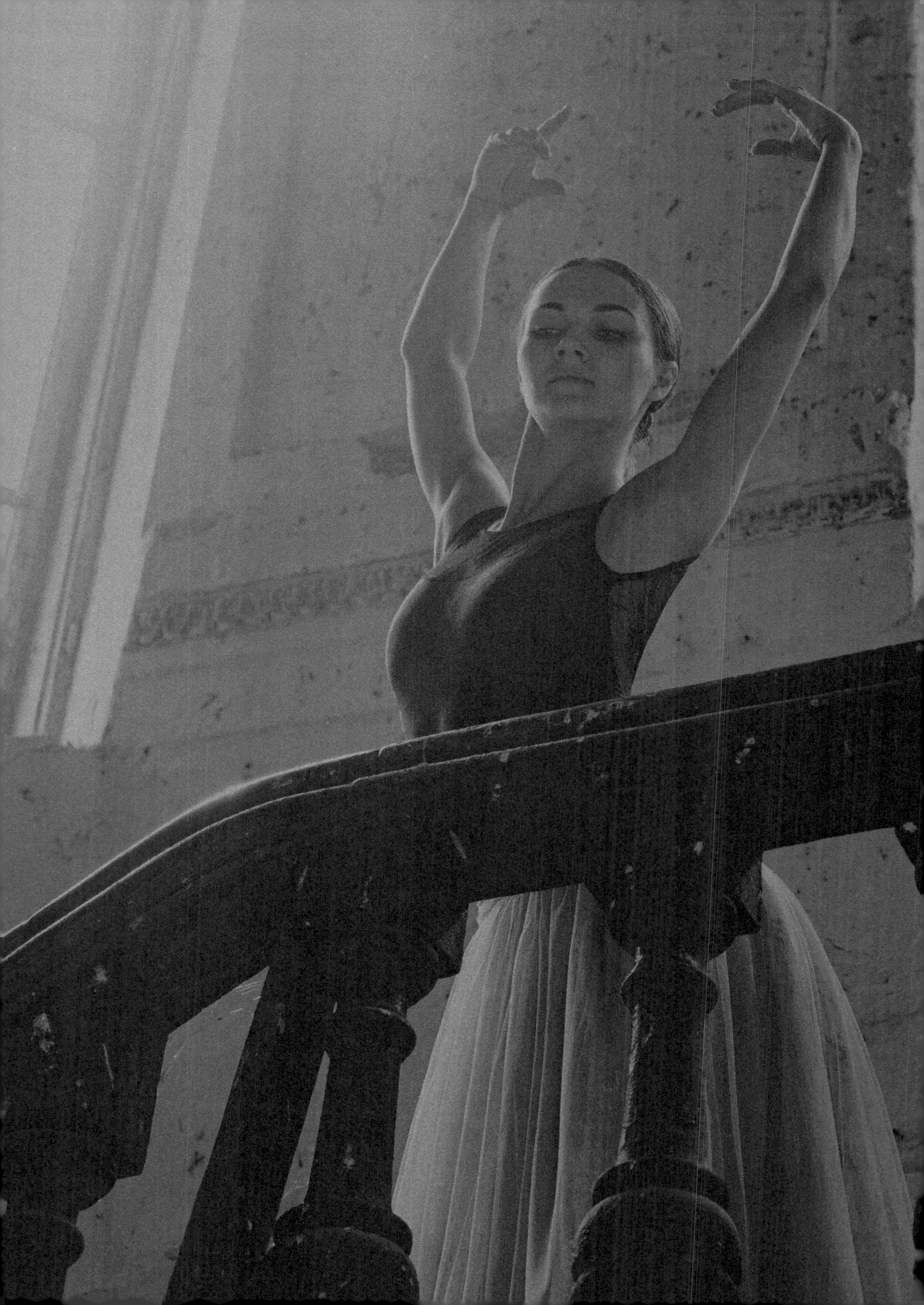

eQUALITY
UNIT #04
'PASSIONS'

The why:
Now we are going to talk about PASSIONS.

There are two types of passions we are interested in. Unit 4 looks at one of them. It is the passion we can't stay away from, something we love to do, that lights up our eyes, gives us energy and makes us feel a sense of purpose and worth.

ACTIVITY 01
THE DIFFERENCE BETWEEN 'PASSION' & 'LIKE'

Read the following and then answer the questions below:

Amy loved craft as a child. When she was twelve, her grandmother introduced her to crocheting.

At first, she did it because she liked being with her gran, but as time went by, she began to love it. She progressed from table mats, to blankets and lacework. She bought a special box to store all the different sized hooks and wools – one she could easily carry and take with her.

As an adult, even when she sits down to watch TV, she crochets. Amy can't imagine going a day without making something.

Jill loved the things Amy, her friend, could make just with one hook and some wool. She thought how relaxing it would be to take up crocheting, to learn a new skill and be able to make something she could use or gift to others.

She bought a set of needles and a varied selection of wool. She bought a couple of books and spent time watching tutorials on YouTube. And for the first few weeks, she spent time every night following patterns, with the intention of making cardigans for her grandchildren.

However, as time went by, she found she had other things to do. She had a busy life, and the crocheting was put off until the next day. Two weeks later, the needles and wool lay in a drawer unused, and, although she thought she ought to pick them up again, she never did.

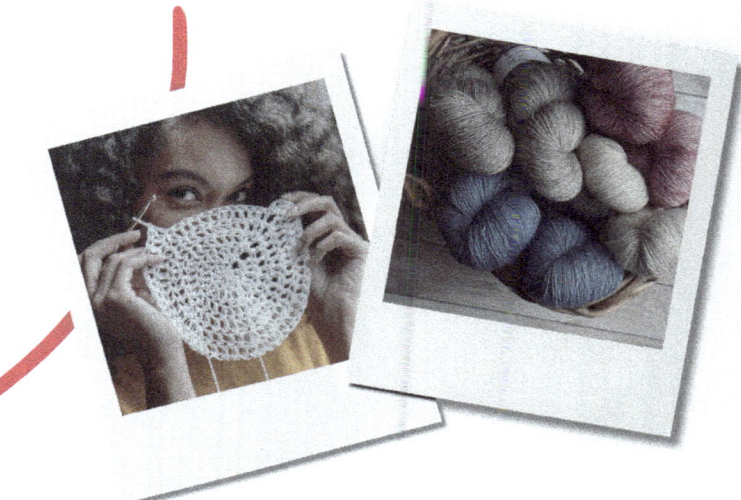

Fill in the questions

Q1. How is having a passion for something different from liking something or just having a whim?

Q2. What does it feel like? What does it look like?

Q3. How does it make you behave?

UNIT 04   'PASSIONS'

ACTIVITY 02
A THOUGHT

> **Do you sometimes stray** towards what others care about, and forget your own dreams, wants or needs?

MY PASSION

WHAT OTHERS CARE ABOUT

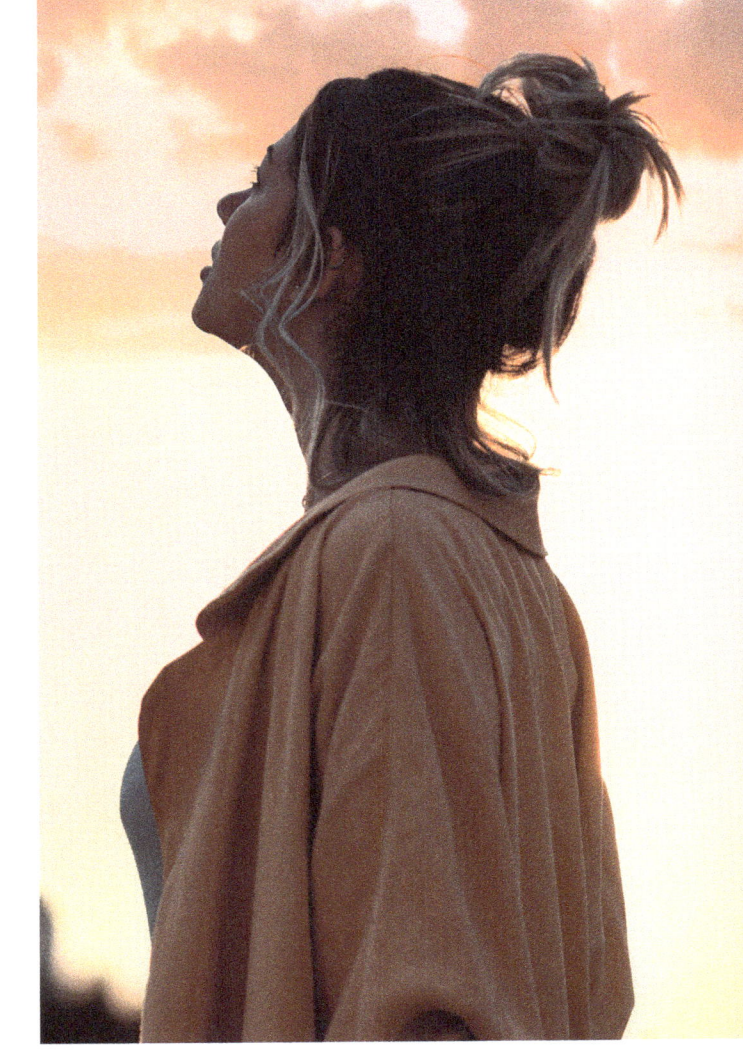

Think about the questions below...

 **01** Why is it important in your life to be aware of our passions?

 **02** How are our passions linked to our likes and strengths?

 **03** How does knowing this affect our careers and future?

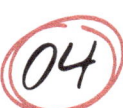 **04** How can it add value to our lives and the lives of others? Is this important?

 **05** Can we use it to make a difference and make a living?

UNIT 04 | 'PASSIONS'

ACTIVITY 03
FINDING YOUR PASSION

Having a passion can give us energy, drive and belief in ourselves. It can help us take steps to achieve. However, some people seem to know what their passions are, others aren't sure. This is normal.

Have a look at the following quiz by Anne Dranitsaris. It may not tell you exactly what your passions are, but it might give you a lead.

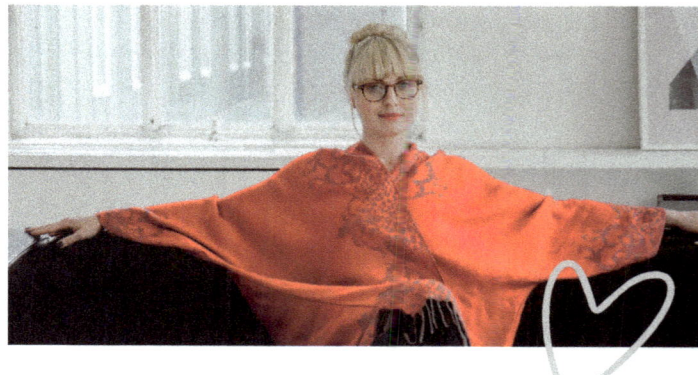

Instructions

You will need a computer or smart phone for this. Search for the below:

> Anne Dranitsaris find your passion quiz

Read each of the statements and ask yourself how true it is for you. Really think about you, not what you think others expect of you. Then rate whether it sounds 'most like you', or 'least like you.' If your first thought when rating a statement is 'it depends', think about how you would react on an average day.

The more honest you are, the more accurate your feedback will be.

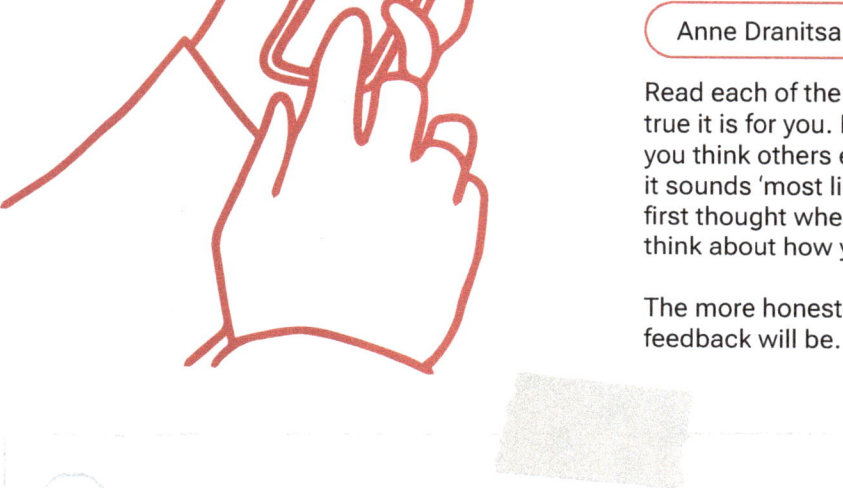

List a few things from the quiz you thought were true or similar to you

_____

_____

_____

_____

'PASSION'
WHAT DOES IT REALLY MEAN?

What does it mean to have a passion about something? The word passion might immediately conjure up images of two people in love, but the word 'passion' has several meanings. The Oxford Dictionary Online describes its meanings below:

 Strong and barely controllable emotion: a man of impetuous passion

 A state or outburst of strong emotion: oratory in which she gradually works herself up into a passion

 Intense love: their all-consuming passion for each other, she nurses a passion for Thomas

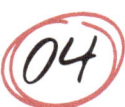 An intense desire or enthusiasm for something: the English have a passion for gardens

 A thing arousing great enthusiasm: modern furniture is a particular passion of Bill's

The type of passion we are talking about here is a combination of points four and five. We are talking about something in your life you could never let go of, that you continually return to, that makes you feel alive and purposeful. It may be a hobby or something more academic, or it may even be a job.

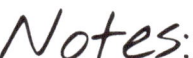

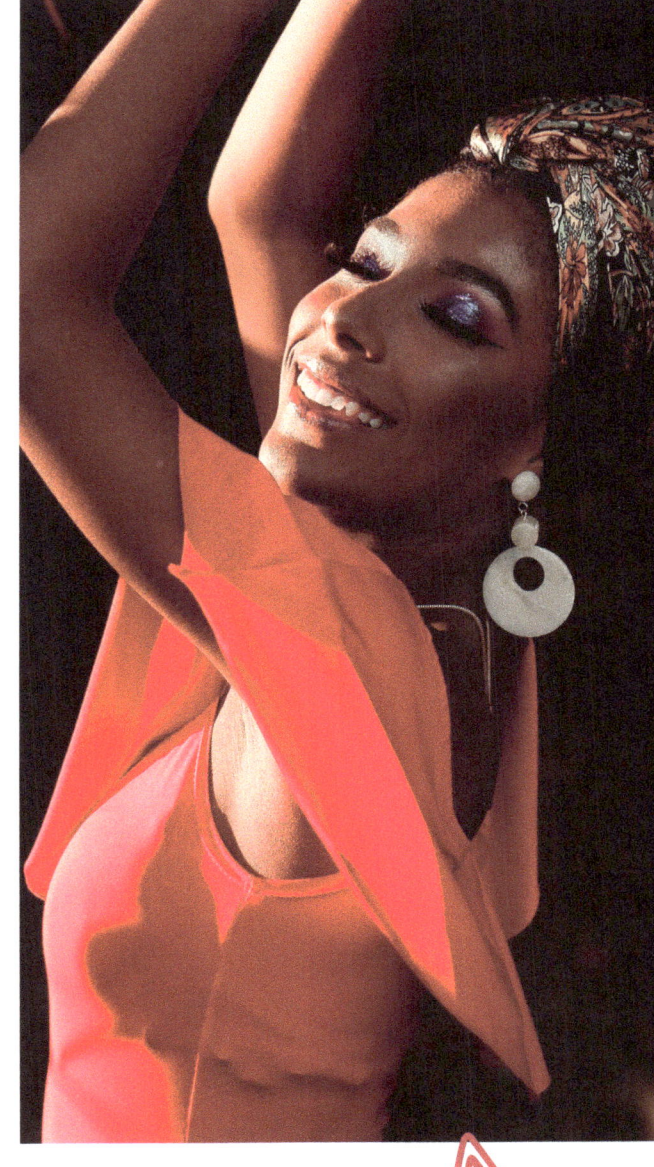

| UNIT 04 | 'PASSIONS' |

REFLECTIONS
YOUR JOURNEY SO FAR

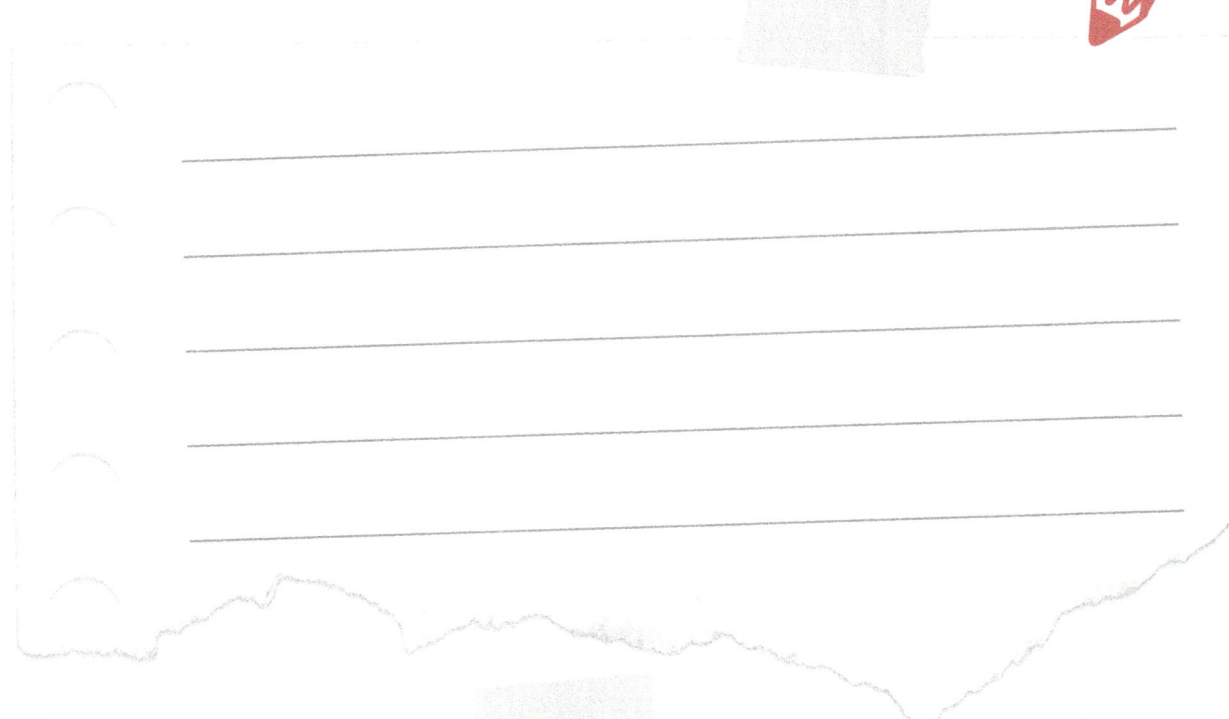

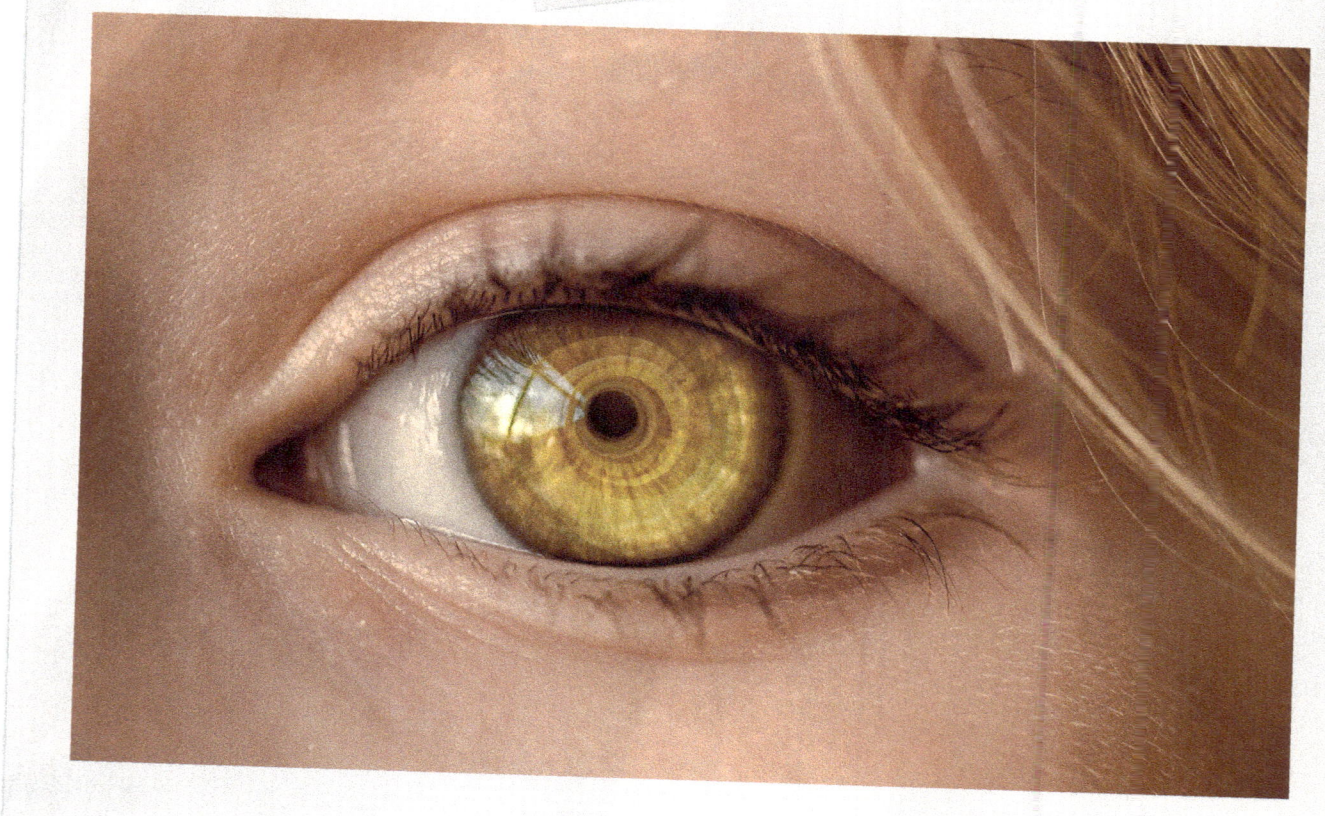

eQUALITY UNIT #05

'DIG OUR HEELS IN'

The why:
It's time to DIG YOUR HEELS IN.

This is the second passion we want to discuss - it relates to principles and personal values. The things we won't compromise on, that may make us dig our heels in or become stubborn. Personal values are usually fairly stable, yet they don't have strict limits or boundaries. As we move through life, our values may change, so understanding them can affect the choices we make, the jobs we pursue or the directions we take in our life.

UNIT 05   'DIG YOUR HEELS IN'

ACTIVITY 01
WHY SO STUBBORN?

> **Read the dialogue below.** It's part of an ongoing discussion between Josie, (aged 13), and her Mum. They are both digging their heels in.

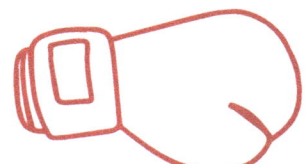
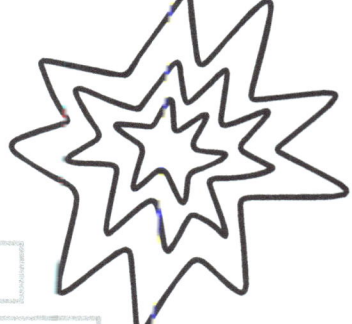

JOSIE	But Mum, I like my room just as it is.
MUM	Josie, this is not under discussion. Clean your room.
JOSIE	Why isn't it under discussion? Can't I say what I think?
MUM	This is nothing to do with that. It's to do with a clean room. Now get on with it.
JOSIE	I'll do it after I finish this game.
MUM	No Josie, you'll do it now.
JOSIE	Why?
MUM	What do you mean, why? Because I asked you to, that's why!
JOSIE	So, I have to do everything you say, when you say it?
MUM	Yes, you do. Get on with it.
JOSIE	So, now this is a dictatorship.
MUM	How dare you speak to me like that young woman? When you have a house of your own, you can keep it as dirty as you like, but right now, you'll do as I say... and not look at me like that. Don't you have any respect?
JOSIE	Why should I respect a dictator?
MUM	Right, for that, you won't be playing any video games for three days.
JOSIE	What?

What's going on here? Why can't they agree?

| UNIT 05 | 'DIG YOUR HEELS IN' |

ACTIVITY 02
WHAT MAKES YOU 'DIG YOUR HEELS IN'?

 **Fill in the smaller circles with different examples of events that have happened**, (either recently or in the past), which have bothered you, so much so that you dug your heels in.

For example, a dog being treated badly by someone, possibly a colleague or friend not pulling their weight, or maybe a sibling not helping with family responsibilities.

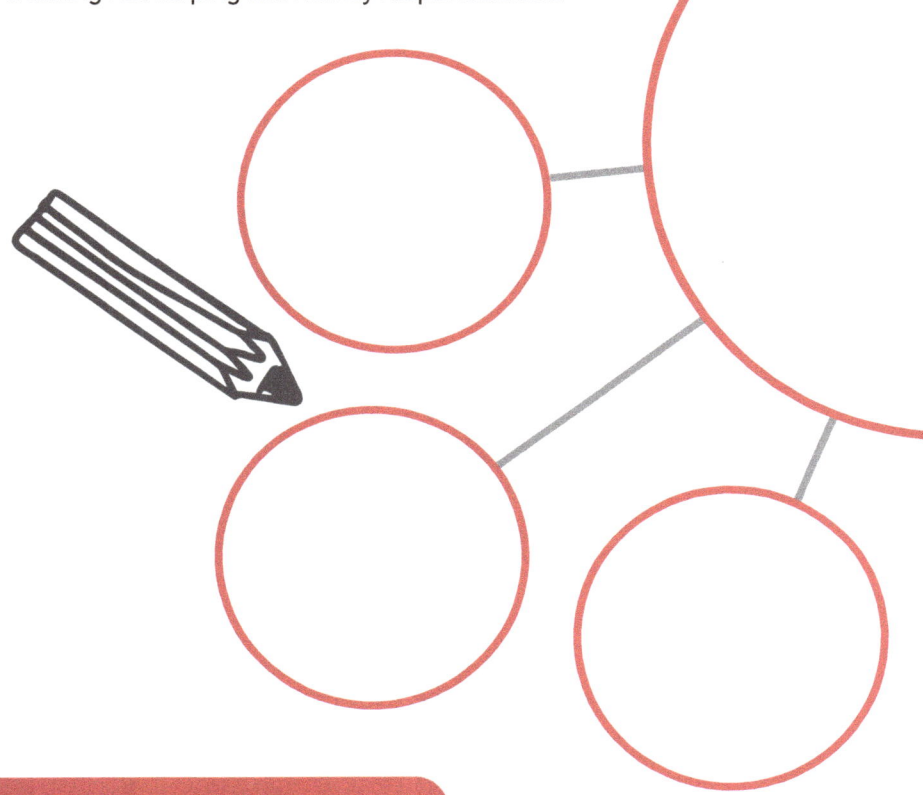

 **Think about the themes that run through each incident.**

Ask yourself;
A. Why did this event make me dig my heels in?

B. Why did I go through the hassle of being difficult?

C. Why in this situation didn't I agree with that person?

Write the themes in the large circle at the top.

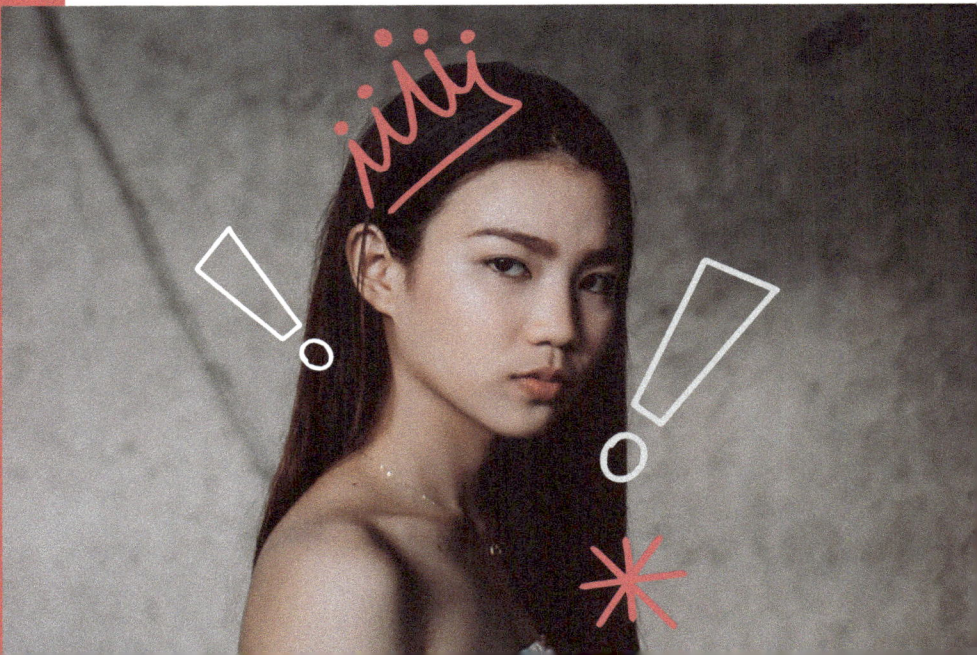

| UNIT 05 | 'DIG YOUR HEELS IN' |

03 Now answers the questions below:

A. Is there anything that has always made you to dig your heels in? (Perhaps a position you always defend.)

B. Do you have a very strong opinion about something that you would not compromise on?

C. Why do you think this happens? How and why might you want to control your reaction?

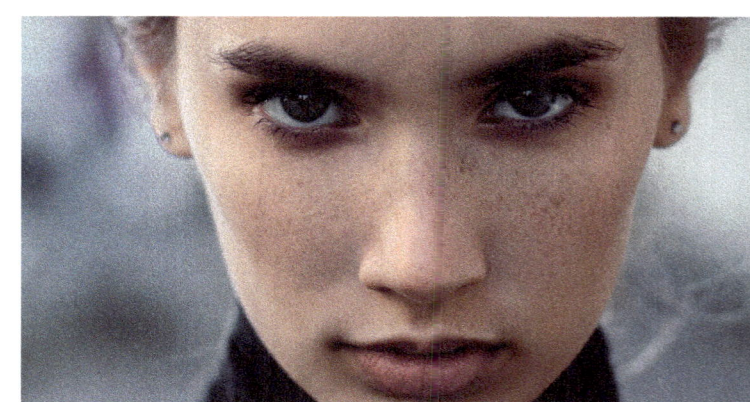

04 Use Activities 1, 2 & 3 as a guide to help you complete the table below:

ISSUE	YOUR REACTION	WHY?

UNIT 05 | 'DIG YOUR HEELS IN'

ACTIVITY 03
PRINCIPLES & PERSONAL VALUES

Both principles and personal values can most often be seen when you dig your heels in on a point, become determined over something and occasionally this may lead to being upset or angry. You may even make a value judgement, 'it's not right', without really understanding why.

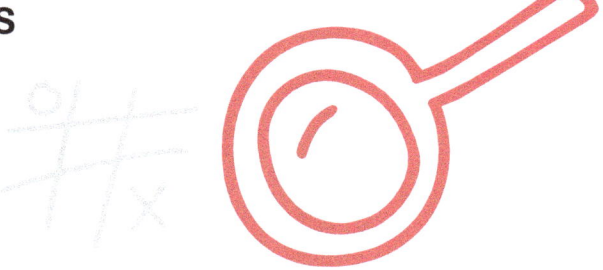

A general truth that many people may hold	A statement that shows our system of beliefs
PRINCIPLES	
A belief that affects our reasoning	From which we may behave in a certain way

Which of the following statements most resonates with you?

- All humans are born equal and should have equal rights, opportunities and a fair justice system.
- Always do the right thing!
- Always live by the highest standards of integrity and honesty.
- Every human being, regardless of gender, age, ethnic origin or creed, is unique and valued.
- Do unto others as you would have them do unto you.
- Do no harm!

ACTIVITY 04
PRINCIPLES & PERSONAL VALUES

VALUES

- A personal view of what is important in life at any one time
- Values are usually fairly stable, yet they don't have strict limits or boundaries
- As you move through life, your values may change
- Understanding them can affect choices you make, how you judge others and which jobs you pursue

Sample personal values

KINDNESS	DETERMINATION	FAIRNESS	HONESTY
RELIABILITY	GENEROSITY		FAITH/HOPEFULNESS
TRUSTWORTHY	FORGIVING	INTEGRITY	COMPASSIONATE
AUTHENTICITY	OPEN-MINDEDNESS		RESPECT
LOYALTY	HUMBLENESS	COURAGE	LOVING

Q1. Think of a time or moment in your life when you were most happy. What made you so happy at the time?

Q2. Write out the things you have done in life you are most proud of, independent of what others thought.

Q3. If you suddenly won the lottery, what would you do next in your life?

Q4. Write about three characters/people, dead, alive, or imaginary, whom you secretly admire. What about them do you most admire?

UNIT 05 — 'DIG YOUR HEELS IN'

ACTIVITY 05
BACK TO YOUR eQUALITY CHART

Complete the third circle in your chart. Instert the things you have a passion about both the positive and the things you feel strongly about that drive you to dig your heels in. You may use objects, pictures, photos, videos, audio or text.

3rd circle

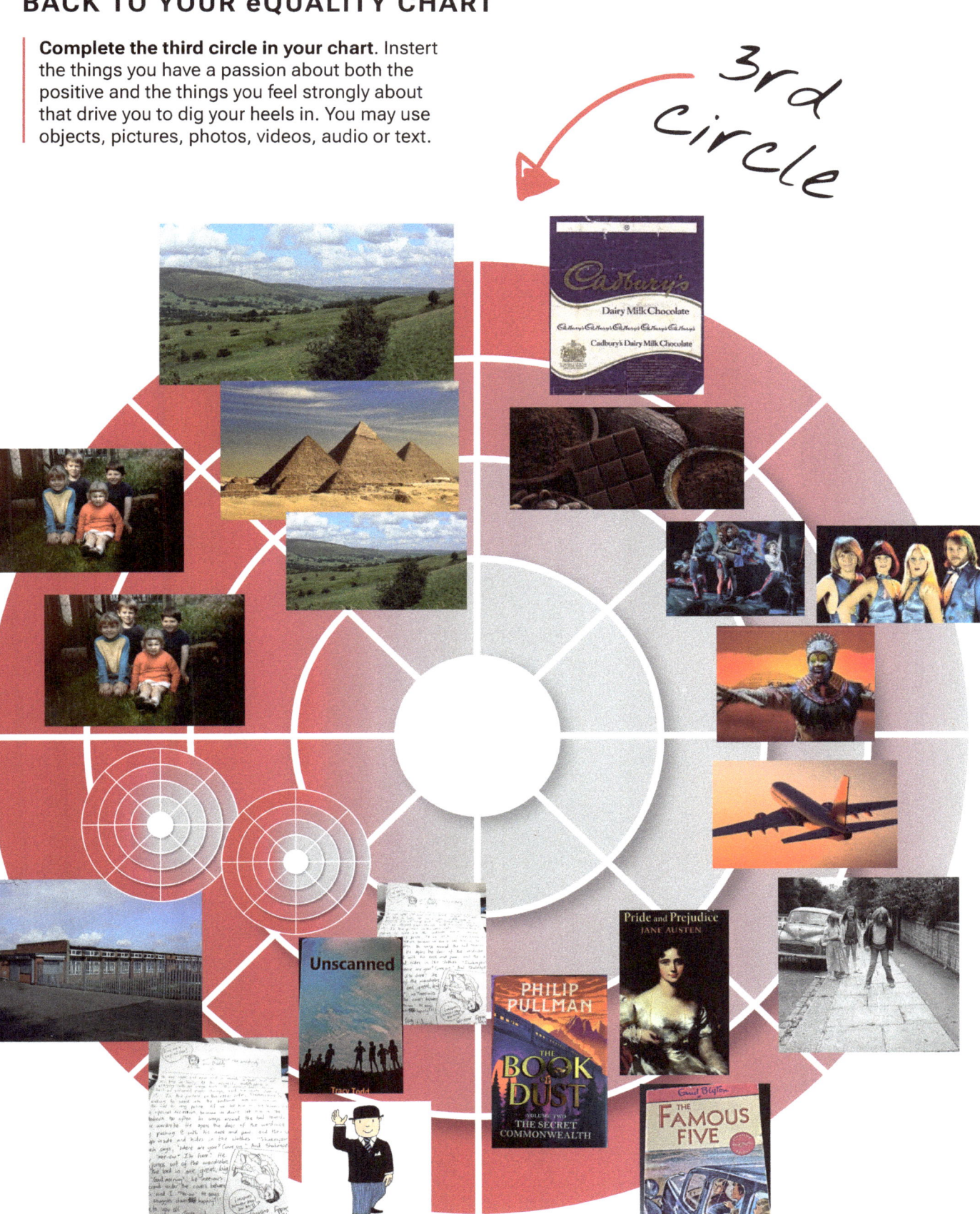

UNIT 05 — 'DIG YOUR HEELS IN'

REFLECTIONS
YOUR JOURNEY SO FAR

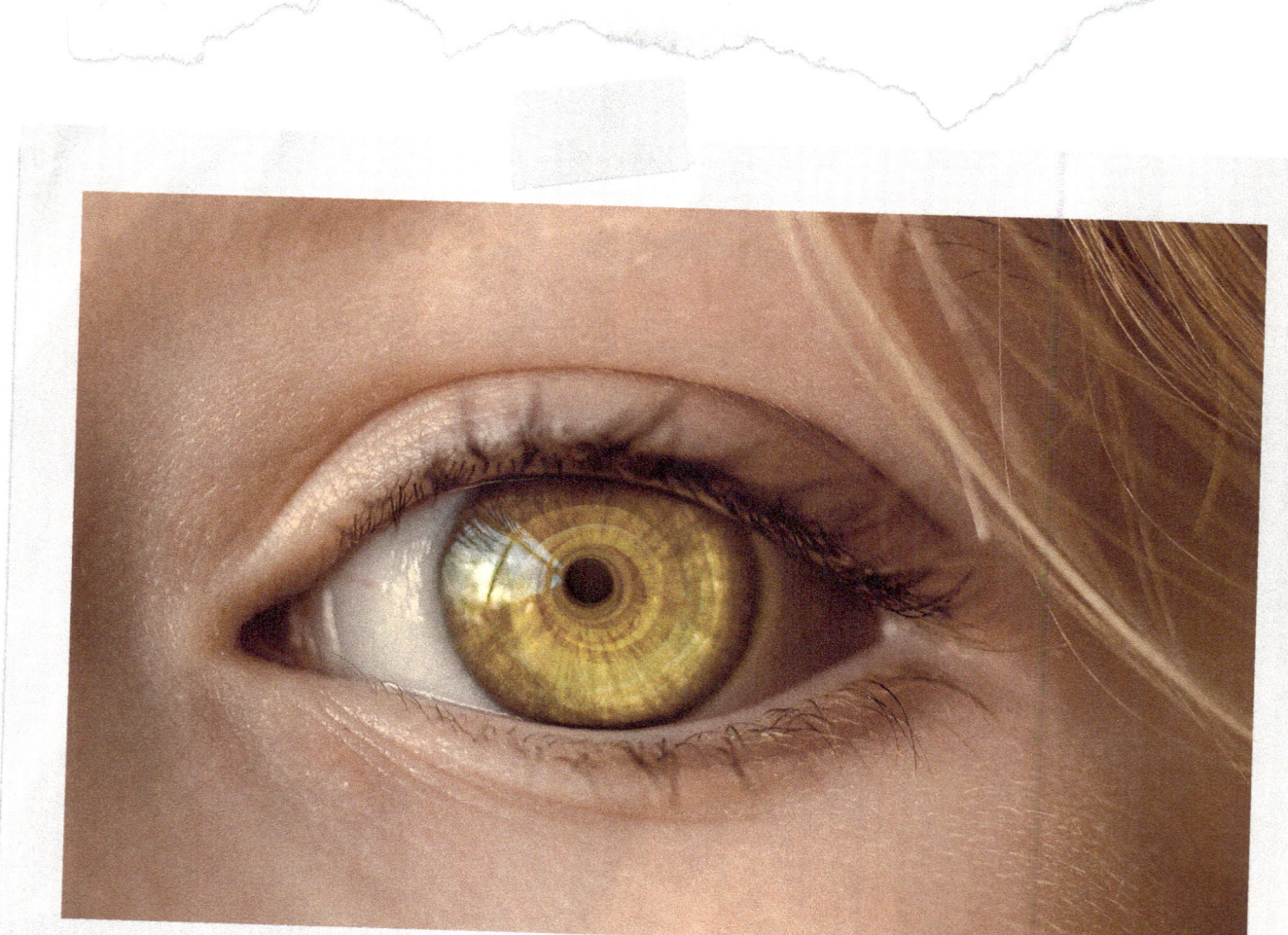

eQUALITY
UNIT #06
'MINDSET'

The why:
Let's take a look at MINDSET

Mindset is a complex set of beliefs, feelings and attitudes we have towards ourselves, those around us and society in general. It can affect how we behave, how we react to things and what we achieve in life. Understanding our mindset and how we can influence it, is a step towards - well let's say - "we step into our power!" In this unit, we discover how to recognise our mindset and know it is a choice.

UNIT 06　　　　　　　　　　　　　　　　　　　　　'MINDSET'

ACTIVITY 01
YOU ARE BEAUTIFUL!

Take a look in the mirror, Ignore the image/reflections. Look into those eyes. Who are you and what can you do? What have you achieved so far? Can you see your beauty now?

Now write down in the mirror below at least five things you like about you.

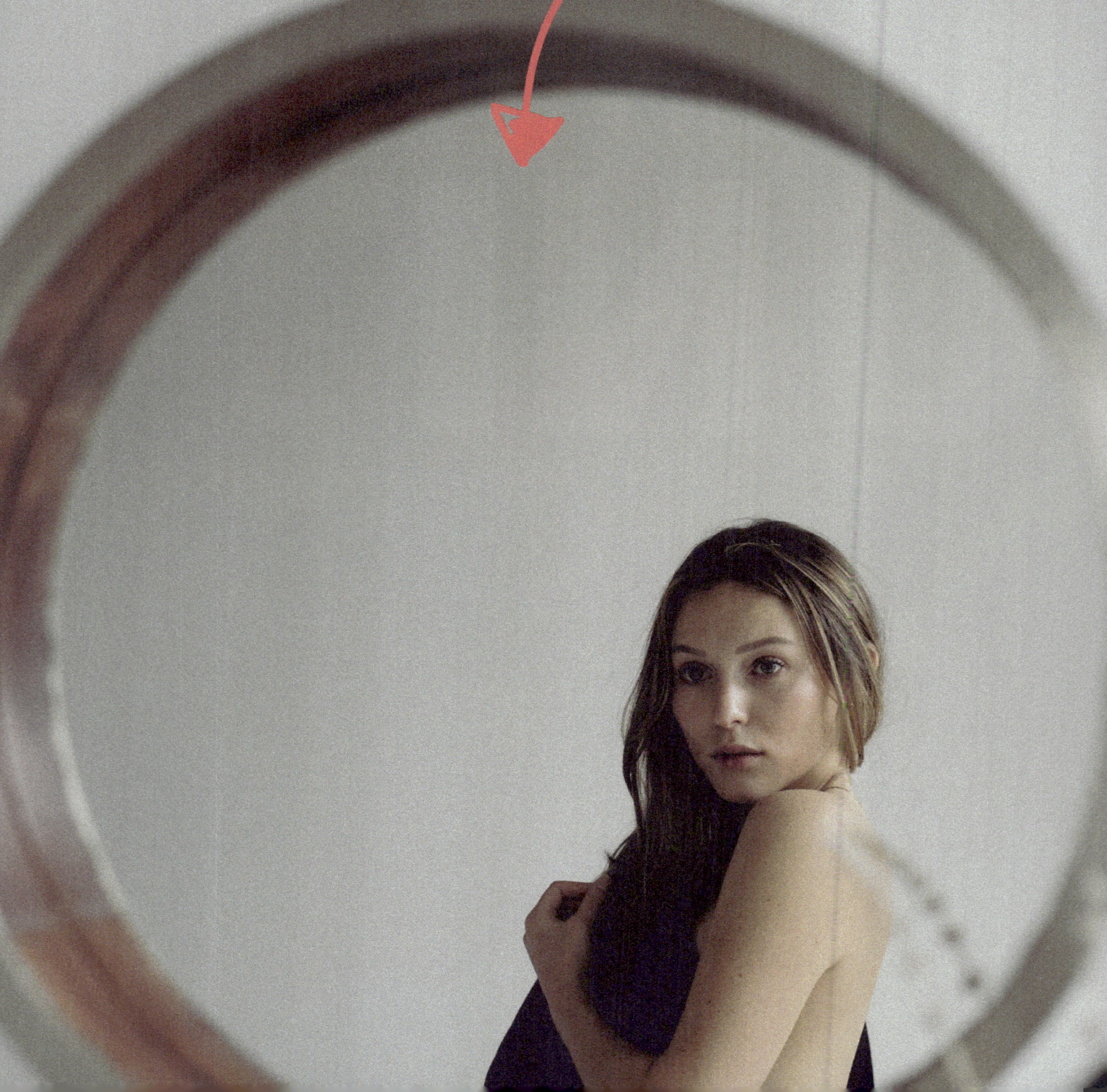

UNIT 06 'MINDSET'

WHAT IS MINDSET?
MINDSET EXPLAINED

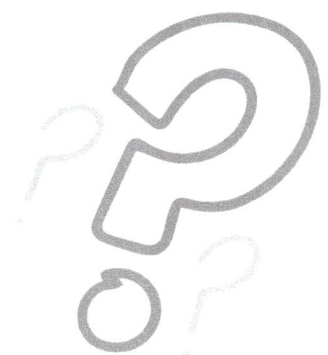

MINDSET

A collection of **thoughts** and **beliefs**

THAT AFFECTS

How you **think**, what you **feel** and what you **do**

RESULTING IN

How **you see yourself** and how you believe **others** see you

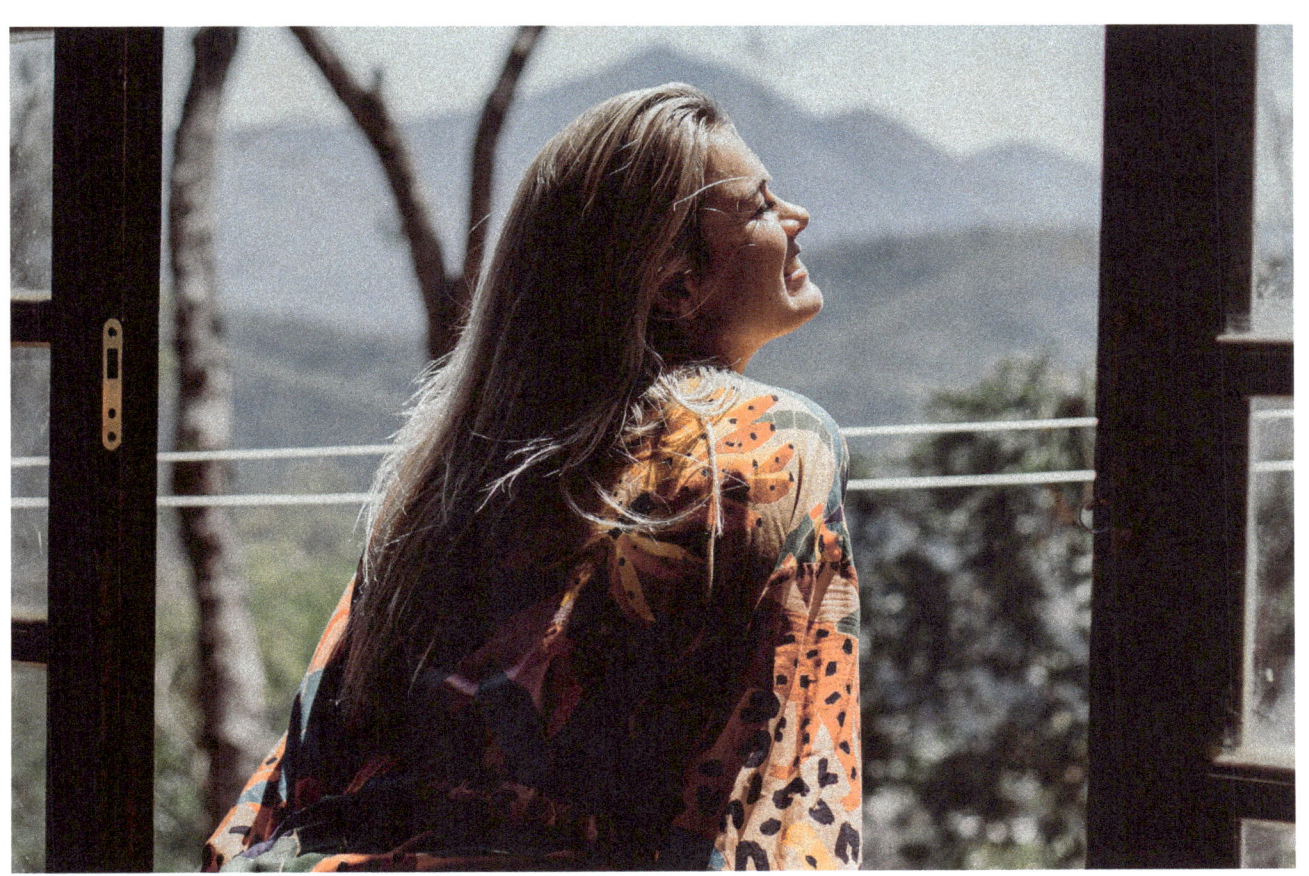

49

UNIT 06 — 'MINDSET'

TYPES OF MINDSET
FIXED VS GROWTH

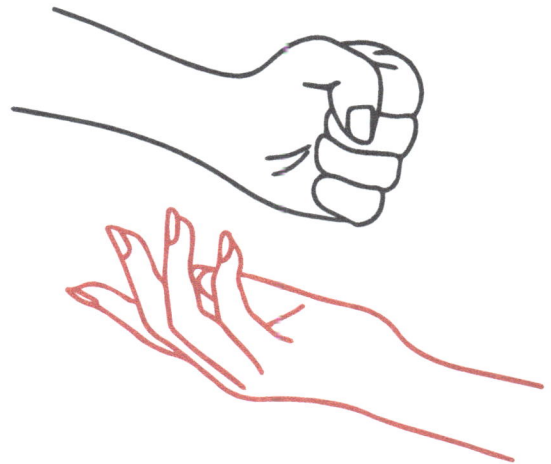

FIXED		GROWTH
The belief that skills, intellect and talents are set and unchangable		The belief that skills, intellect and talents can be developed through practice, perseverance and continual learning
I'll stick to what I know. Either I'm good at it or not.	**DESIRES**	I want to learn new things. I am eager to take risks.
It's fine the way it is. There is nothing to change.	**SKILLS**	Is this really my best work? What else can I improve?
This is a waste of time, there's a lot to figure out.	**EFFORT**	I know this will help me even though it is difficult.
It's easier to give up. I'm really not smart.	**SETBACKS**	I'll use another strategy, my mistakes help me learn.
This work is boring. No one likes to do it.	**FEEDBACK**	I recognise my weakness, and I know what I want to fix.
It's easy for them. They were born smart.	**TALENTED PEERS**	I wonder how they did it. Let me try to figure it out.

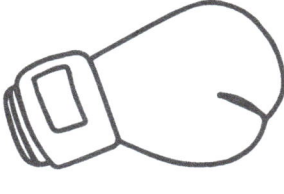 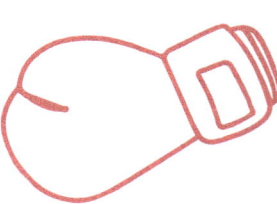

CHANGING MINDSET
3 STEPS TO CHANGING YOUR MINDSET

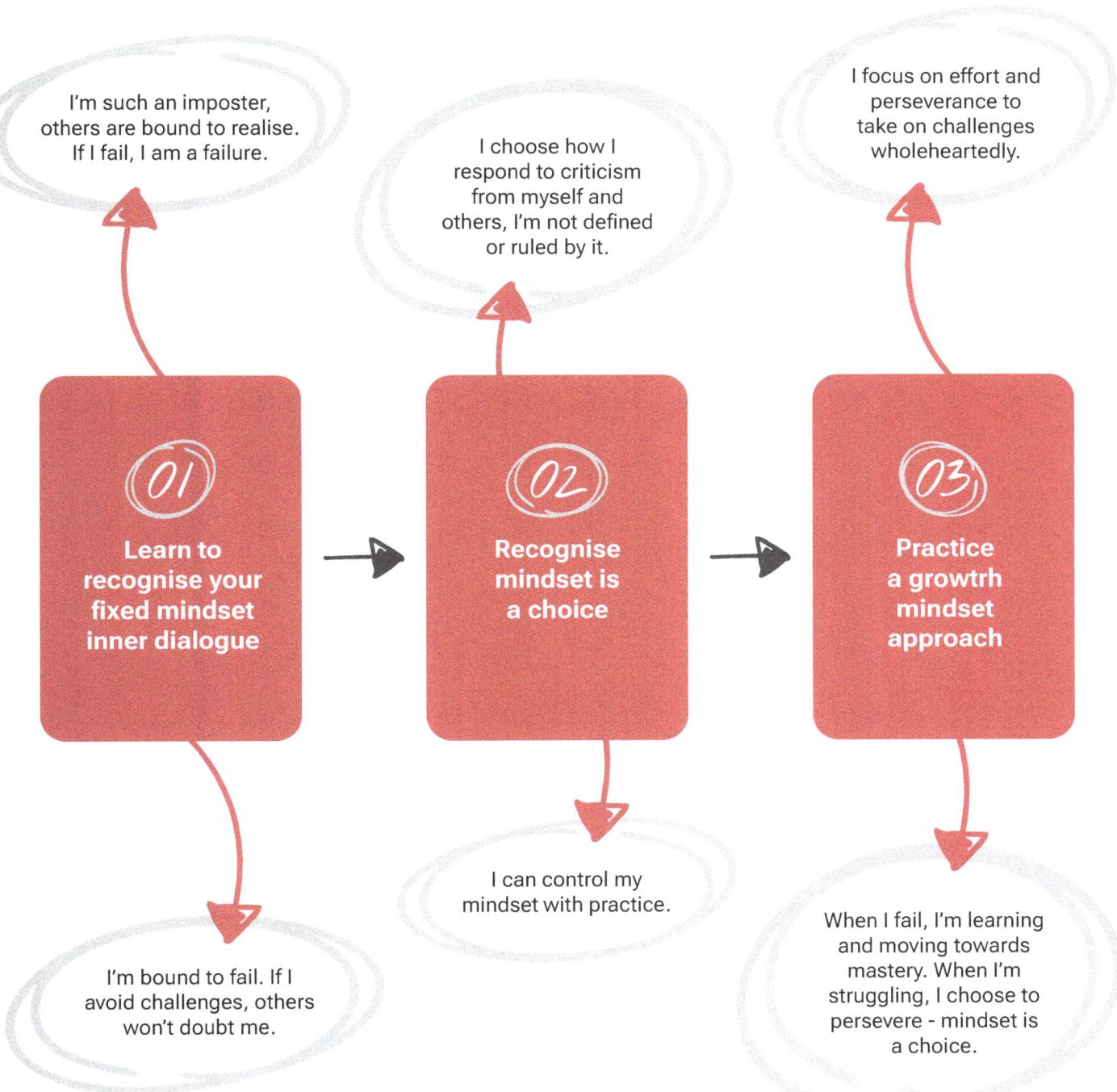

ACTIVITY 02
GROWTH MINDSET BOX

Read the Growth Mindset Chart below with a trusted friend. Discuss which sentences you hear yourself saying to yourself most regularly and which you are ready to change.

If there are none here that relate to you, what do you say to yourself that needs flipping?

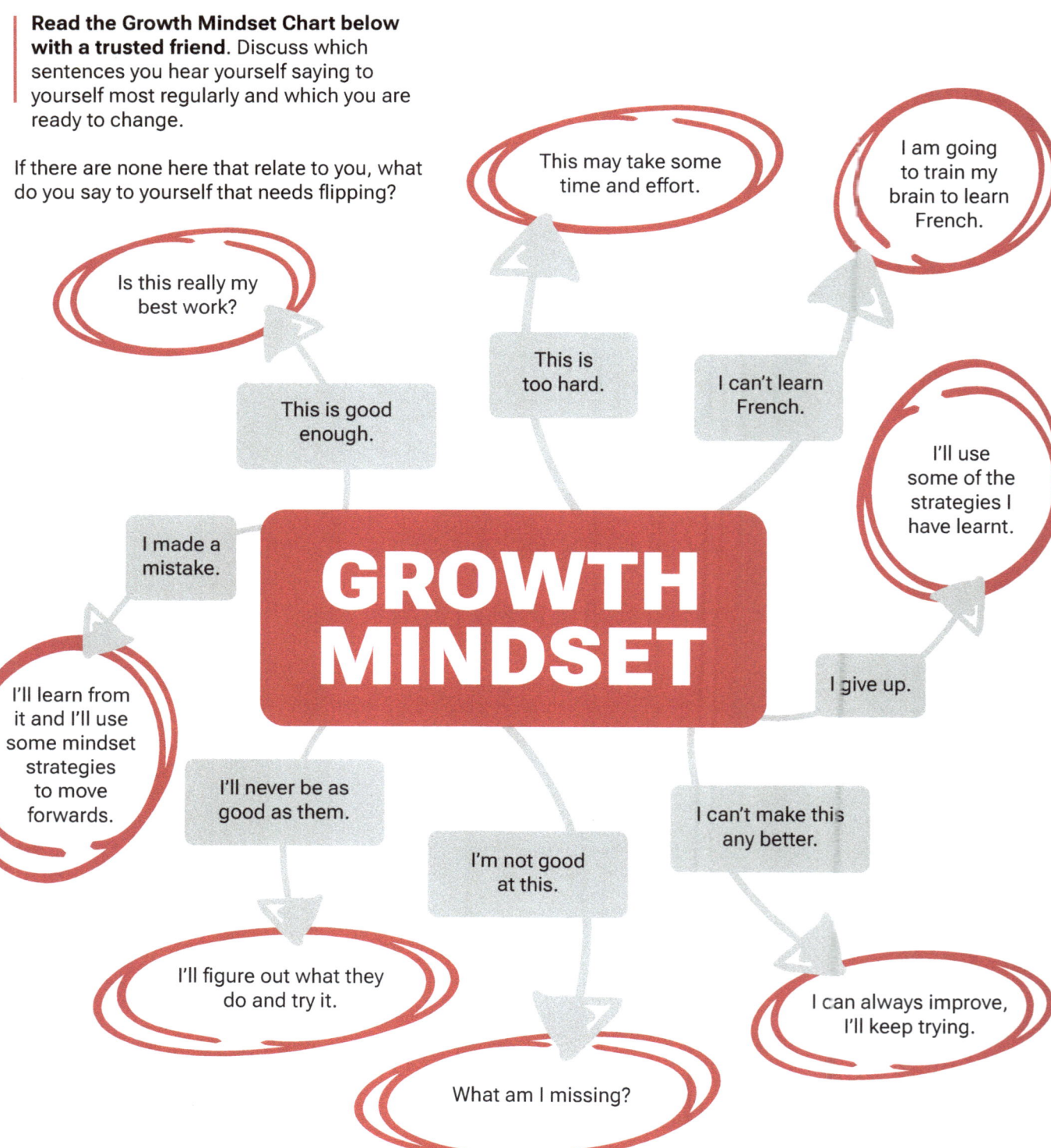

| UNIT 06 | 'MINDSET' |

FLIP THAT *negative* VOICE.

MAKE A COMMITMENT TO YOURSELF

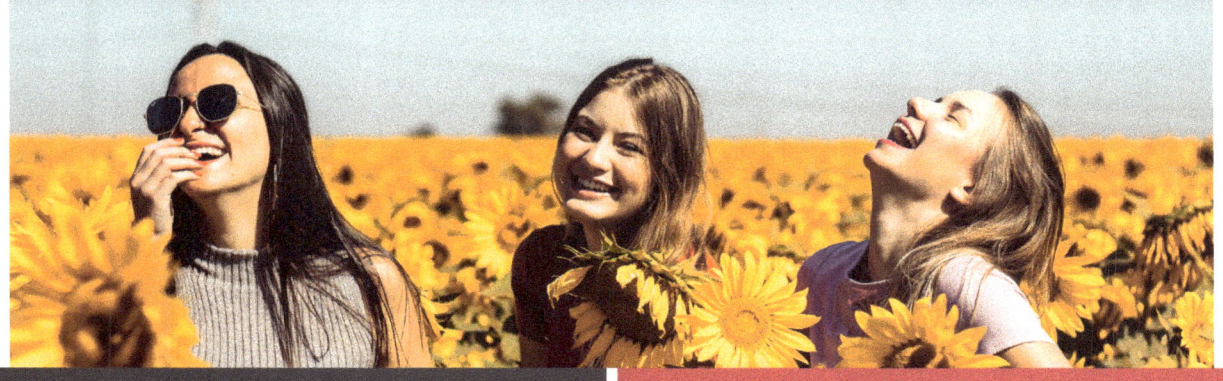

IF I HEAR THIS ▶ **I WILL SAY THIS**

| UNIT 06 'MINDSET'

ACTIVITY 03
RECOGNISE YOUR POWER

Think of a time when you felt confident and experienced a sense of self-worth.

Answer the questions

Q1. How would you describe the situation? What happened?

Q2. What did you say to yourself about the situation (self-talk)? What tone did your self-talk have? What kind of language did you use?

Q3. What physical sensations and feelings were you aware of?

Q4. What did you do or what happened, as a result of this?

What have you learnt about yourself during this activity?

UNIT 06   'MINDSET'

CONFIDENCE
FEEL GOOD ABOUT YOURSELF

Confidence is one of the keys to feeling good about ourselves and loving the person we are and who we are becoming.

We can make an effort to feel confident in who we are and what we can achieve, although it can take time.

We have to remind ourselves that we're an amazing person and that we deserve to feel good about ourselves.

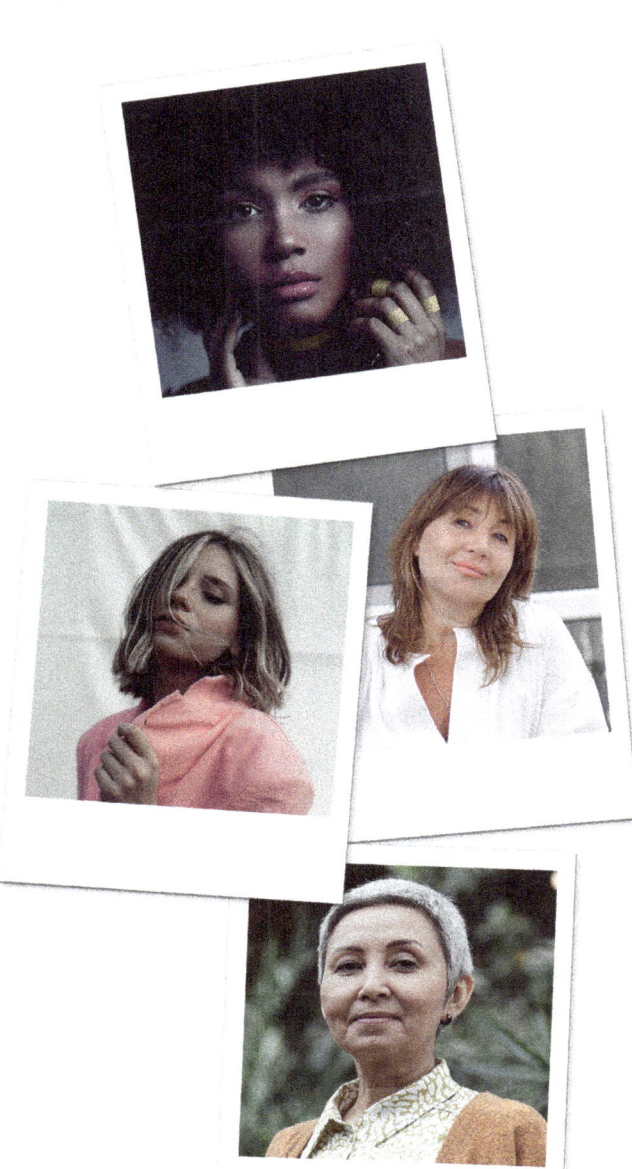

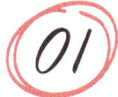 01 — Take ten deep breaths

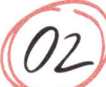 02 — Smile

 03 — Appreciate yourself

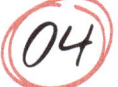 04 — Meditate

 05 — Spend time with loved ones

 06 — Go outside. Breathe fresh air, walk in the countryside, go to the park

 07 — Put down your phone

 08 — Exercise more

 09 — Learn something new

 10 — Help others

| UNIT 06 | 'MINDSET' |

ACTIVITY 04
GROWTH MINDSET AFFIRMATIONS

1. Mistakes help me learn and grow
2. I haven't figured it out YET
3. I am on the right track
4. I can do hard things
5. This might take time and effort
6. I stick with things and don't give up easily
7. I strive for progress, not perfection
8. I go after my dreams
9. I cheer myself up when it gets hard
10. I am a problem solver
11. I try new things
12. I embrace new challenges
13. Learning is my superpower
14. I am brave enough to try
15. I improve with lots of practice
16. I grow my brain by learning hard things
17. I try different strategies
18. When I don't succeed right away, I try again
19. I ask for help when I need it
20. I learn from my mistakes
21. I focus on my own results
22. I was born to learn
23. When I fail, I say "I can't do it YET" and try again
24. I strive to do my best
25. I can learn anything!

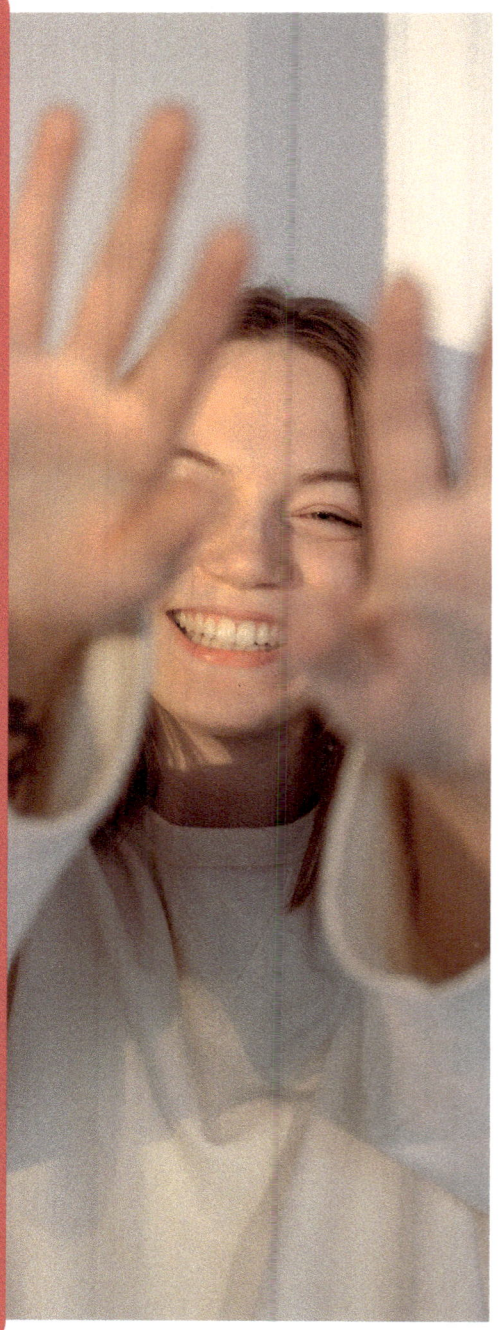

Credit: Big Life Journal - biglifejournal.com

UNIT 06 'MINDSET'

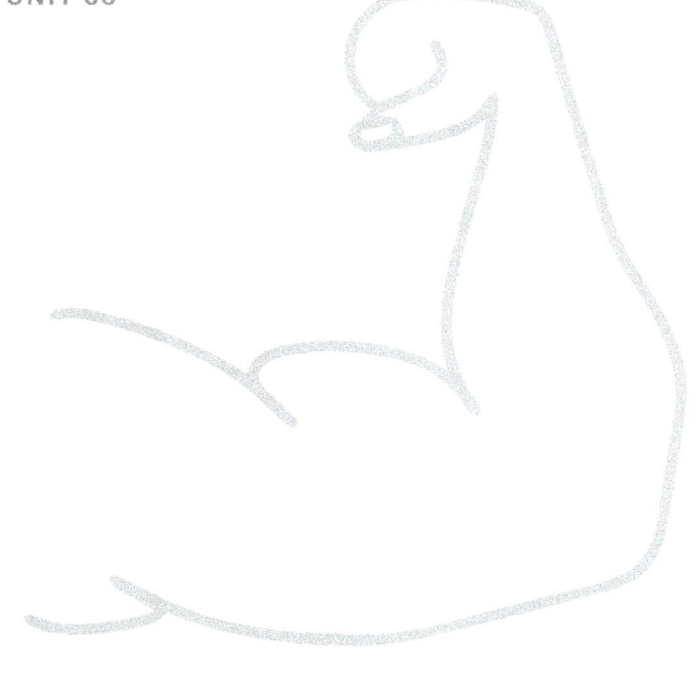

LAURA DING-EDWARDS

WHEN THE WORLD IS ON YOUR SHOULDERS

When the world is on your shoulders
And your heart feels full of lead
And your stomach churns like butter
And the voice inside your head
Is reminding you of everything
You've ever said or done
All your failures and regrets
All the times your fear has won
Take a minute to remember
That you've survived this all before
You've battled and you've conquered
When you thought you had no more
You are stronger than you realise
You are brave and wise and kind
And you know you're so much bigger
Than the doubts that fill your mind
So, breathe it in, then let it out
Allow the ebb and flow
You can win this war, you always do
You're a warrior you know.

| UNIT 06 | 'MINDSET' |

REFLECTIONS
YOUR JOURNEY SO FAR

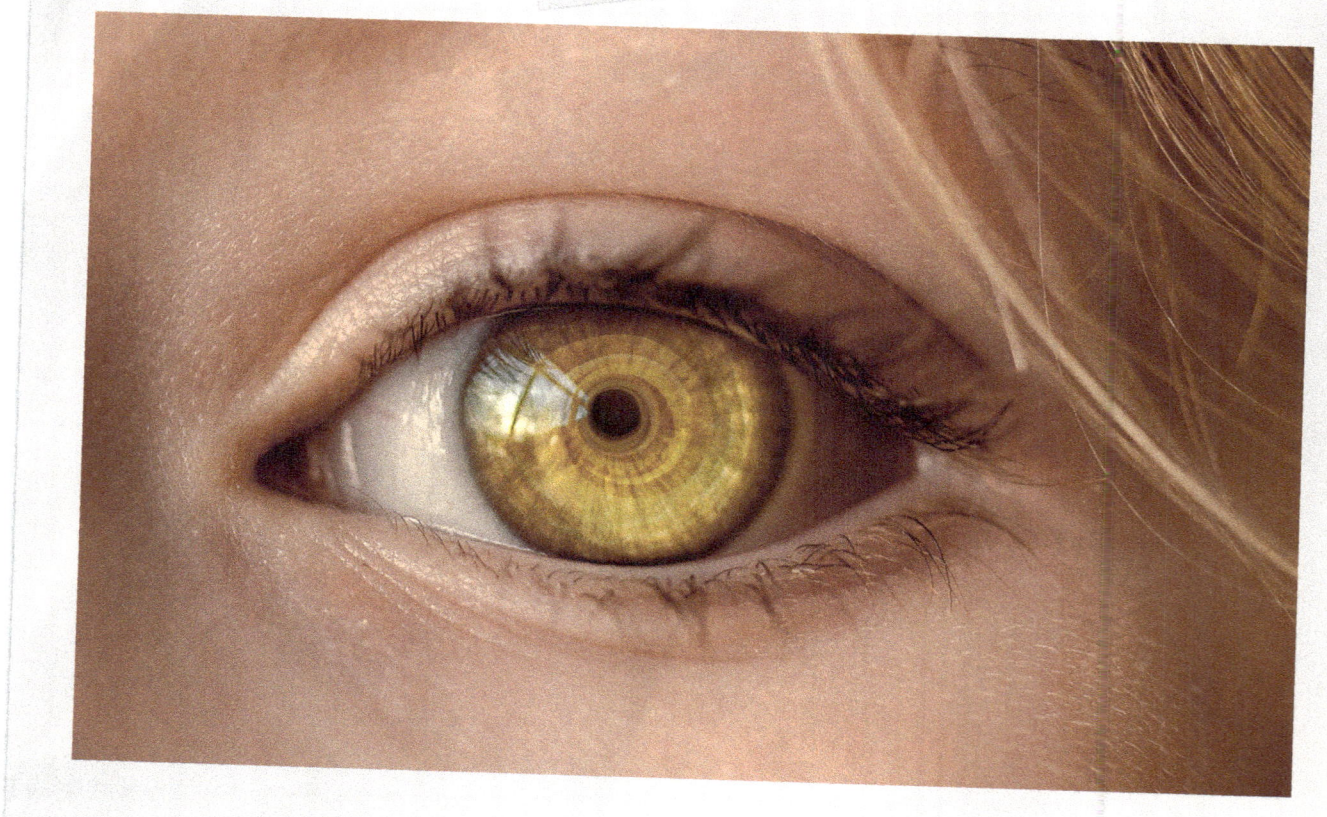

eQUALITY
UNIT #07
'LIFE DREAM'

The why:
Discovering our LIFE DREAM

This unit focuses on discovering our dream life and why knowing what it is, is the most pragmatic first step we can take to feeling more fulfilled and having a sense of purpose.

UNIT 07 | 'LIFE DREAM'

ACTIVITY 01

WHAT IS A 'LIFE DREAM'?

The expression 'Life Dream' is often thought of as silly. People make fun of it. For some, it isn't cool to talk about. You may have been told.

"That's all very well as a hobby, but how are you going to make money? Be practical, you have bills to pay!"

Dreams don't have to lead to being 'rich and famous'. Our dreams belong to us, whatever we want to achieve.

Answer the questions;

1. Who are they?
2. What did they achieve?
3. What do you think their life dreams were?

_____

_____

_____

_____

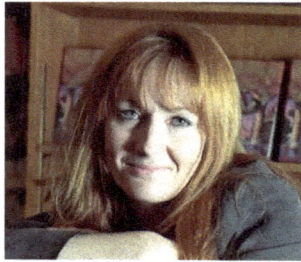 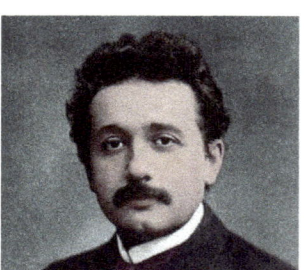 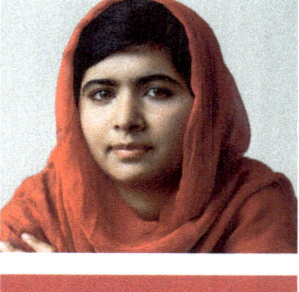 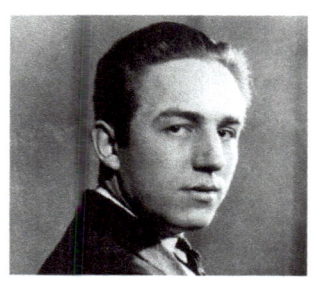

Before this person became rich publishing a series of novels, she was nearly penniless, severely depressed, divorced and trying to raise a child on her own, while attending college and writing a novel. She went from depending on welfare to being one of the richest women in the world in a span of only five years through her hard work and determination.	This person didn't always show such promise. He did not speak until he was four and did not read until he was seven, causing his teachers and parents to think he had a learning disability, because he was slow and anti-social. He was expelled from school, but eventually won the Nobel Prize and changed the face of modern physics.	This person was born 12 July 1997 in Pakistan and became an early advocate for girl's education. At just 15, she was shot after taking an exam by the Pakistani Taliban, which caused international outrage. She was brought to England to recover and founded the Masala Fund for girls. She also co-authored 'I Am Masala', which became an international best seller. Later she went on to receive the 2014 Nobel Peace Prize.	This person made billions from merchandise, movies and theme parks around the world, but he had a bit of a rough start. He was fired by a newspaper editor because, 'he lacked imagination and had no good ideas'. After that, he started a number of businesses that didn't last too long and ended in bankruptcy and failure. He kept plugging away, however, and eventually found a recipe for success that worked.

See the end of the unit for the answers.

UNIT 07   'LIFE DREAM'

ACTIVITY 02

WHO DO YOU KNOW?

Do you know someone that has a life dream and is struggling to achieve it? What is it? What are they doing?

_____
_____
_____
_____

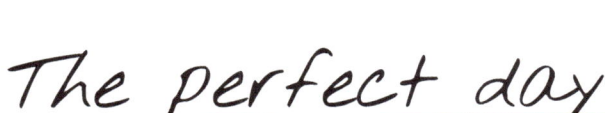

When we're children, it's easier to have dreams. 'I want to be an astronaut.' 'I want to be a singer.'

As we get older, we can lose that sense of 'anything is possible', and often don't even know what our perfect day looks like.

Can you remember what your perfect day looked like when you were a child?

TIME	ACTIVITY
09:00 - 11:00	ICT
11:00 - 11:15	Maths
11:15 - 11:30	English
11:30 - 11:50	BREAK
11:50 - 12:50	Apparatus Work
12:50 - 13:30	Lunch Break
13:30 - 15:30	Science
15:30 - 16:30	Football
16:30	END OF DAY

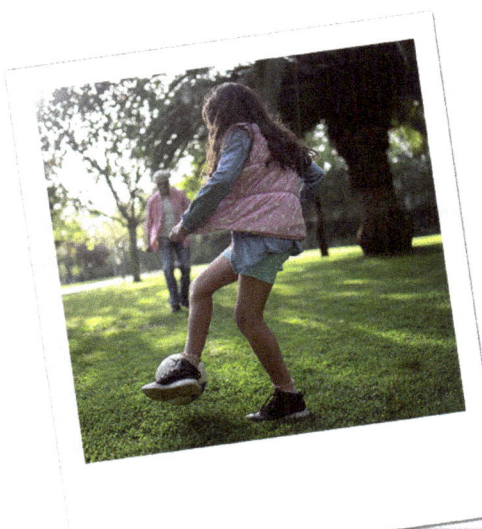

| UNIT 07 | 'LIFE DREAM' |

ACTIVITY 03
YOUR PERFECT DAY

Think about your perfect day now and fill in the table below. Think of things you'd actually like to achieve, things that interest you... not just having a cup of tea or lunch with friends.

This is not a day at the spa, more a work day. A day when you achieve. What is your perfect work day?

TIME	ACTIVITY

If you really could have this day just as you planned it, how would it make you feel? Describe your feelings. Put one or two words in each of the circles below.

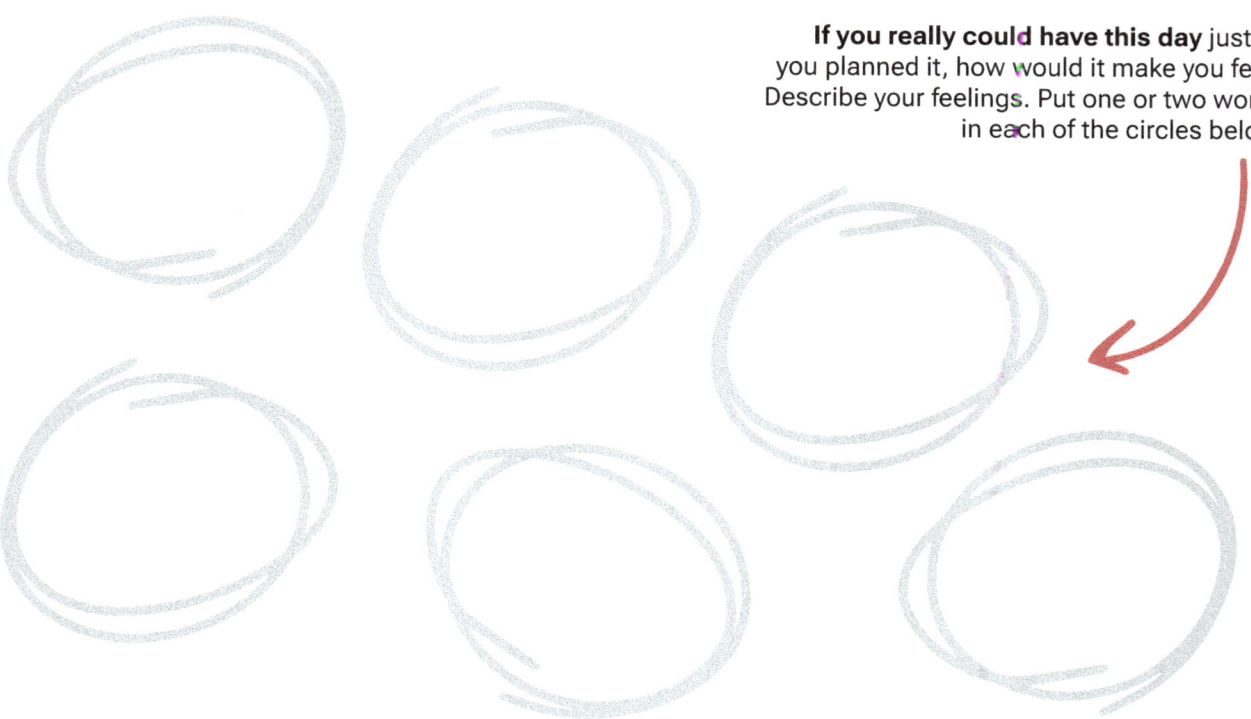

UNIT 07 'LIFE DREAM'

ACTIVITY 04
LET'S GET STARTED

Consider the questions. Think about your answers and jot down some notes.

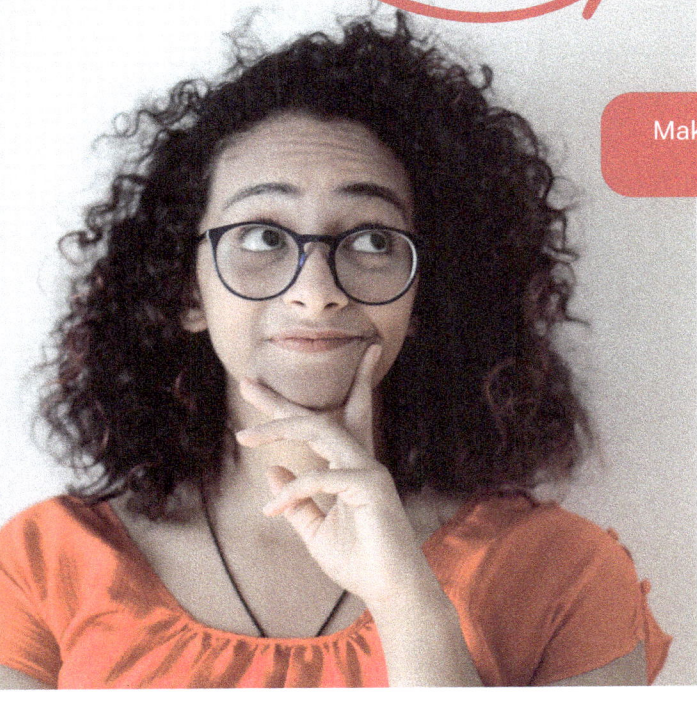

- If you haven't already, start by listing all the things you like/have a passion for in order of preference.
- Ask yourself: what/who would I work with, i.e. people, animals, machinery etc.
- Make a 'bucket list': Everything you would like to do if no one judged you and you had a billion pounds.
- Think about what could make you forget to eat or go to the toilet.
- Ask yourself, how is my one life going to make a difference to me and to others?
- What would you like people to remember you for when they walk away?

UNIT 07 'LIFE DREAM'

ACTIVITY 05
IF YOU HAD TO...

LEAVE HOME **ALL DAY** **EVERY DAY**

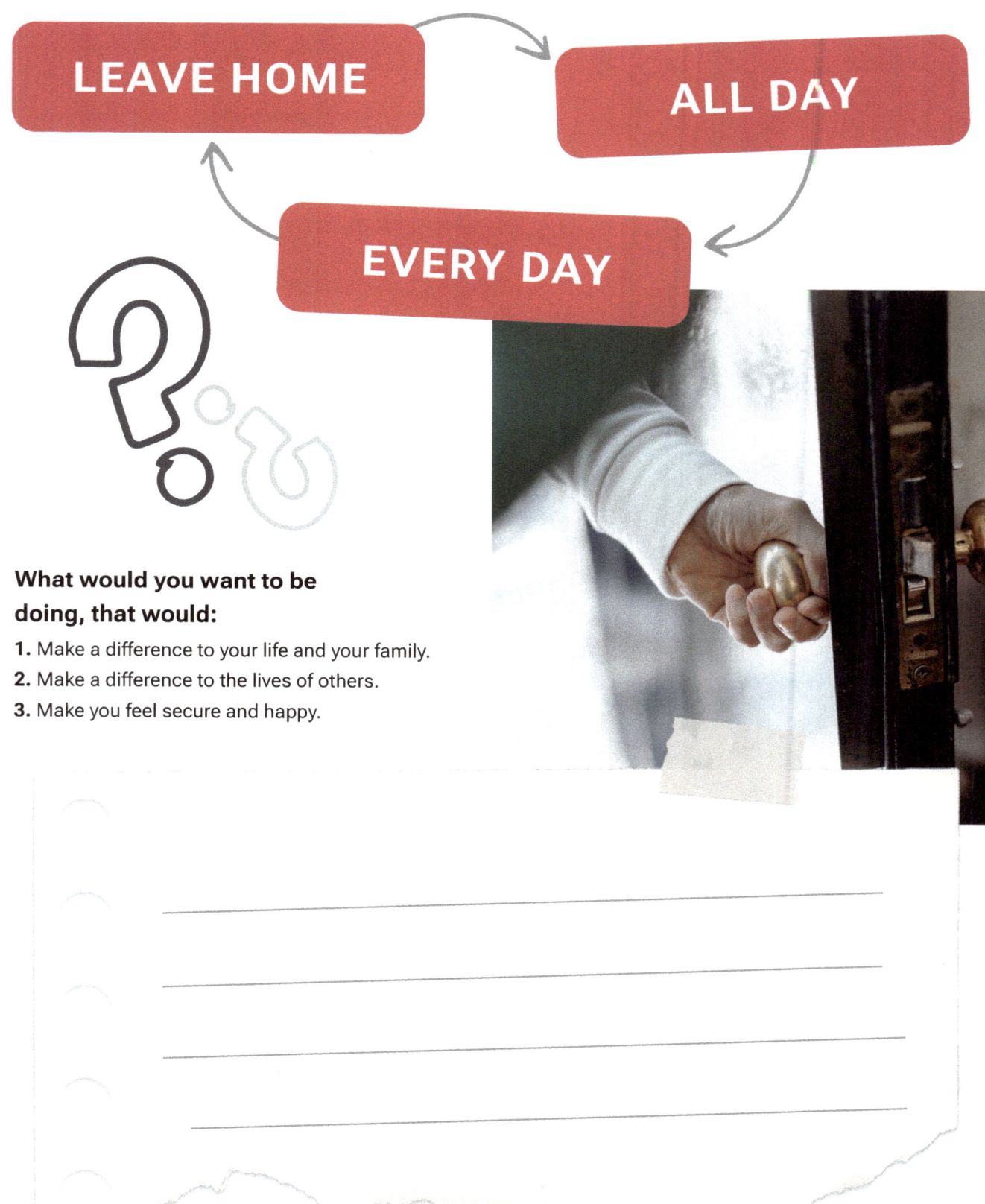

What would you want to be doing, that would:

1. Make a difference to your life and your family.
2. Make a difference to the lives of others.
3. Make you feel secure and happy.

UNIT 07   'LIFE DREAM'

ACTIVITY 06

TRAITS OF AN IDEAL EMPLOYEE

> **Forbes,** a top American business magazine, listed its top fifteen traits of an ideal employee. Here are some of them:

- SUCCESSFUL
- AMBITIOUS
- PASSIONATE
- HARD WORKING
- DETAIL FOCUSED
- INTELLIGENT

Forbes International stated: You can train an employee on your product or service, but you can't train someone to have integrity, resiliency, self-confidence and work ethic.

[Forbes 15 traits of the ideal employee]

So, will a person following their life dream be an ideal employer? Will they believe in what they are doing, be passionate, ambitious to achieve, hard-working and detail/action-focused?

SO, IS A LIFE DREAM PRACTICAL?

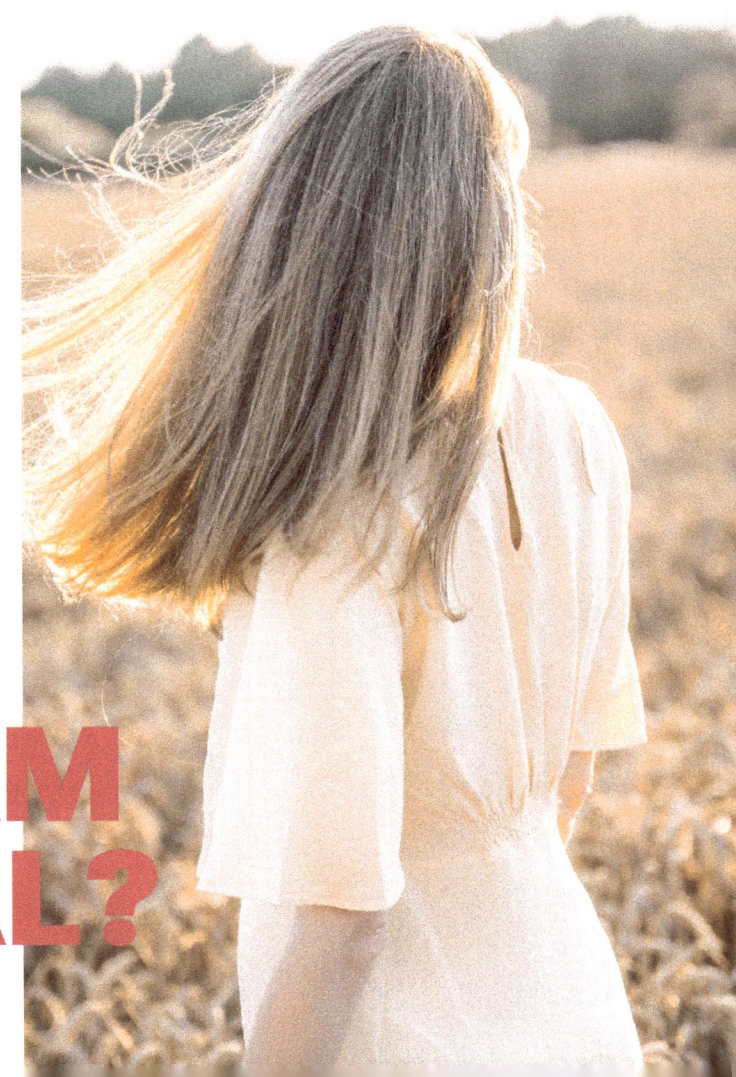

ACTIVITY 07
BACK TO YOUR eQUALITY CHART

Complete the fourth circle of your chart. What does your dream life look like, and what might you be doing to achieve it. You may use images, photos, videos, audio or text.

4th circle

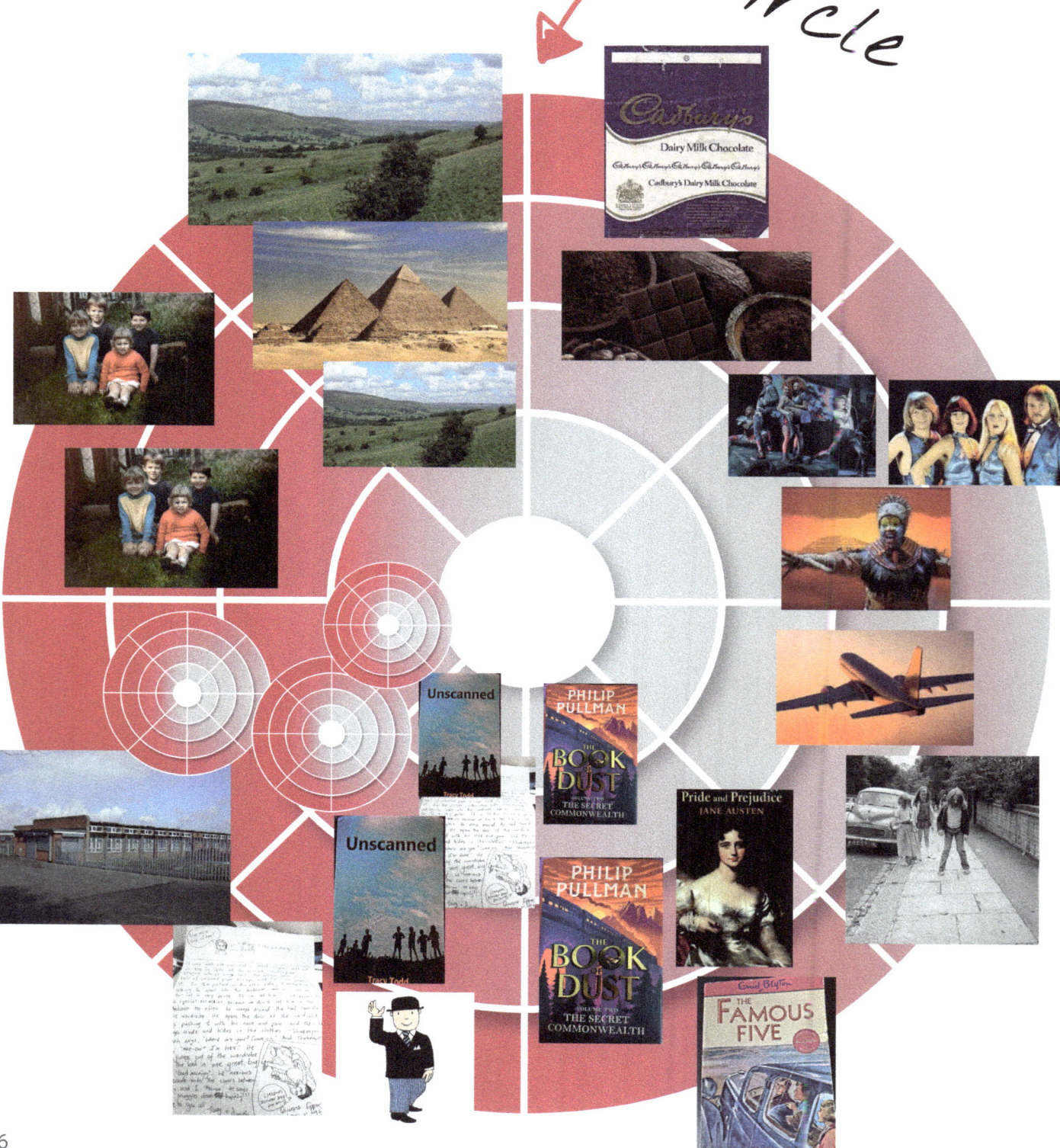

| UNIT 07   'LIFE DREAM' |

REFLECTIONS
YOUR JOURNEY SO FAR

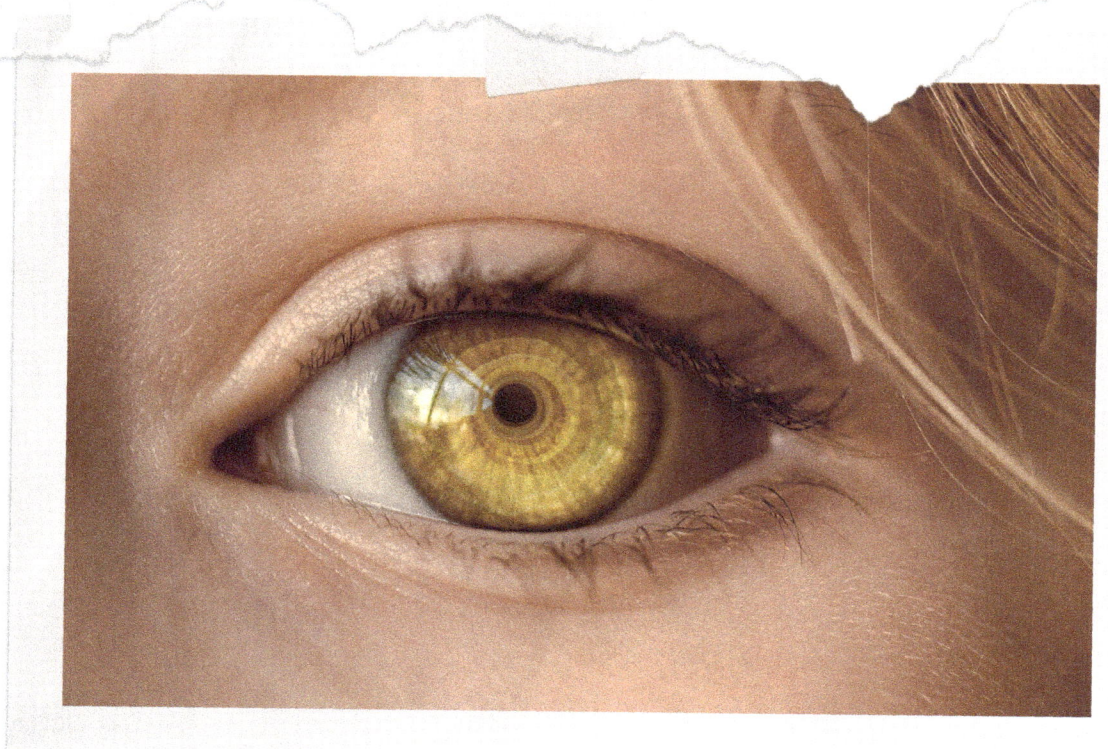

Answers to Activity 21

A: J. K. Rowling, Author of Harry Potter Series.
B: Albert Einstein, Scientist. Most famous for the Theory of Relativity.
C: Malala Yousafzai. Most famous for taking a stand on women's education.
D: Walt Disney. Most famous for the creation of Disney films and theme parks.

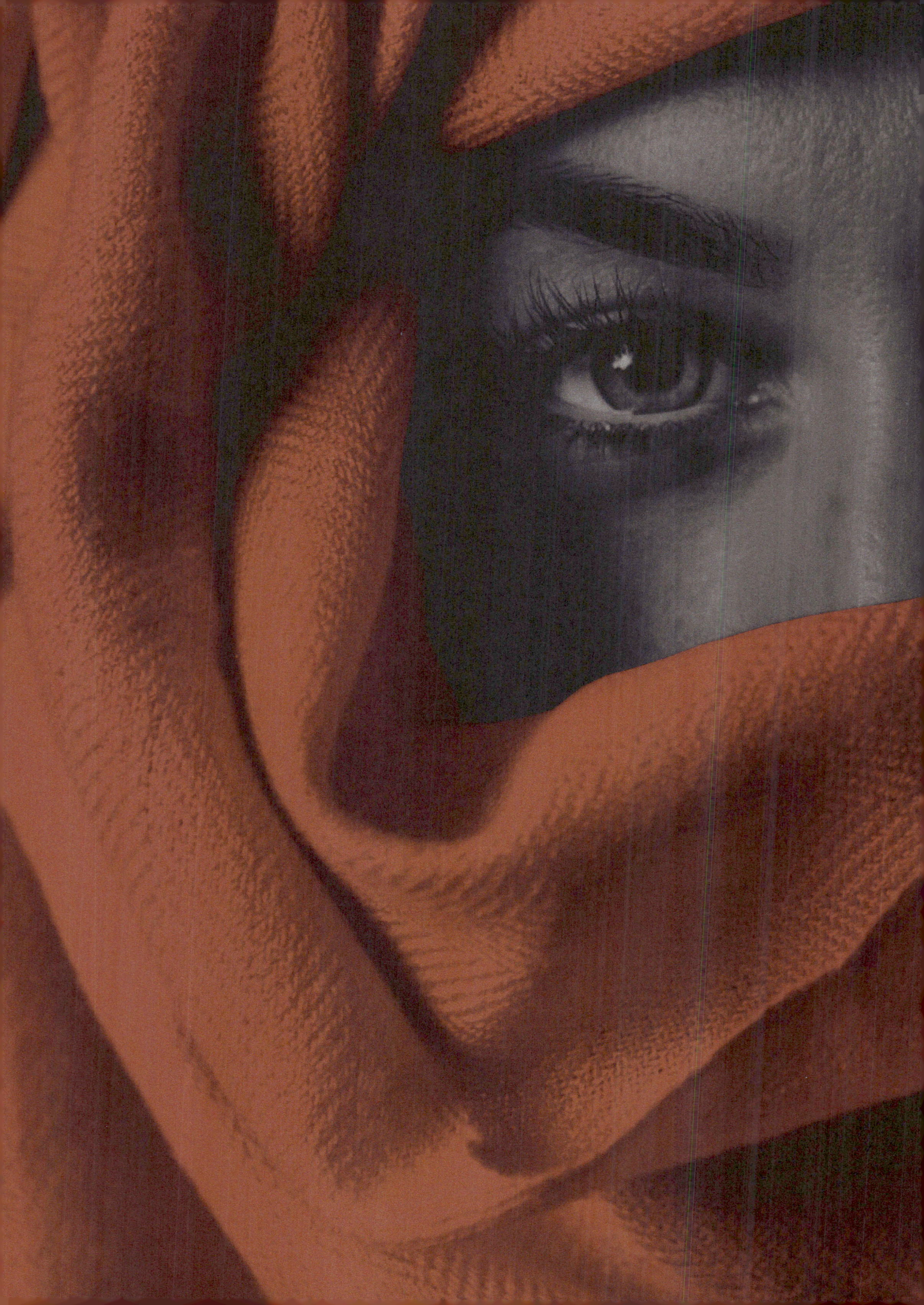

eQUALITY 👀
UNIT #08
'VISION'

The why:
Seeing our VISION.

Vision is about being what we are right now, in the moment. If we can see our vision, feel it and know it, we are already half way to achieving it.

UNIT 08 'YOUR VISION'

ACTIVITY 01
eQUALITY CHART LINKS

What links are you beginning to see in your eQuality Chart? Write down some observations here.

_____
_____
_____
_____

> We all have dreams. But in order to make dreams become a reality, it takes an awful lot of determination, dedication, self-discipline, and effort.
>
> **Jesse Owens**
> **Track Athlete**

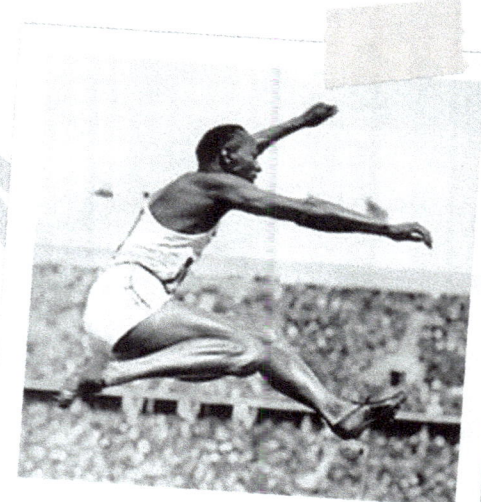

Jesse Owens

ACTIVITY 02
REMEMBER YOUR PERFECT DAY...

What do you do that seems to speed up time?
You might look at your watch and say 'Wow, I've lost an hour. Where did that go?

_____
_____
_____

UNIT 08   'YOUR VISION'

ACTIVITY 03
ENVISIONING

> **Envisioning is about placing yourself in a situation and imagining it happening.** If you can see yourself doing something, it is the first step to making it happen.

The exercise below aim to help you envision your future, based on what your life dream is. Take some time to really think about this.

Imagine yourself five years from now.

You are leaving your home. It's a beautiful Spring day. What are you wearing? The sun is shining, you are heading to your ideal workplace. How are you getting to work? Picture yourself travelling to work, what smells are in the air on this beautiful day? What do you hear? This is your dream job, how does it make you feel to be heading to your dream job?

**You arrive at work.
Where are you?
What are you?**

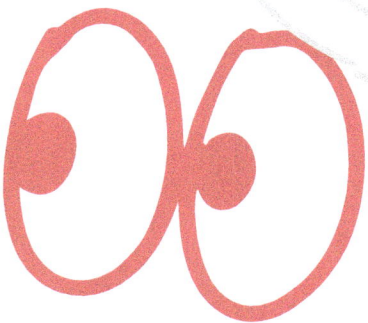

Answer the questions

_____

_____

_____

_____

_____

_____

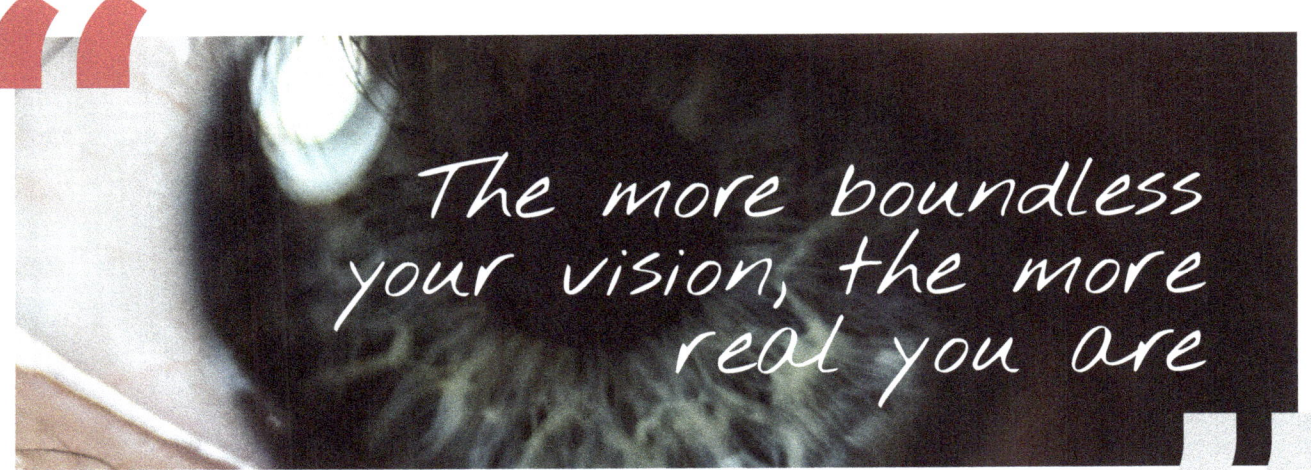

" *The more boundless your vision, the more real you are* "

UNIT 08 'YOUR VISION'

ACTIVITY 04
WRITING DOWN YOUR VISION

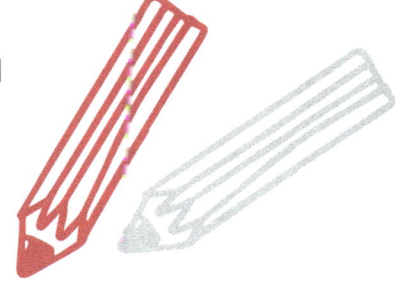

> **Use the present tense:** "I am a...."
> Don't limit yourself or say, 'I can't do that!'

If I say I can or I say I can't, I'm probably right!

EXAMPLE " I am a recognised writer, giving children all over the world pleasure in the written word.

I AM A...

BY WHEN?

Is it one year, five years, ten years from now? Give an estimated number of years:

YEARS

Review of your eQuality Chart

PAST LIKES | CURRENT LIKES | PASSIONS | DREAM LIFE | VISION

UNIT 08   'YOUR VISION'

ACTIVITY 05
DEVELOPING A VISION

Developing a vision is the first step to achieving your dream life. Writing it down and telling people about it, is the second step!

The chart below sums up some of the strengths you need to achieve your vision.

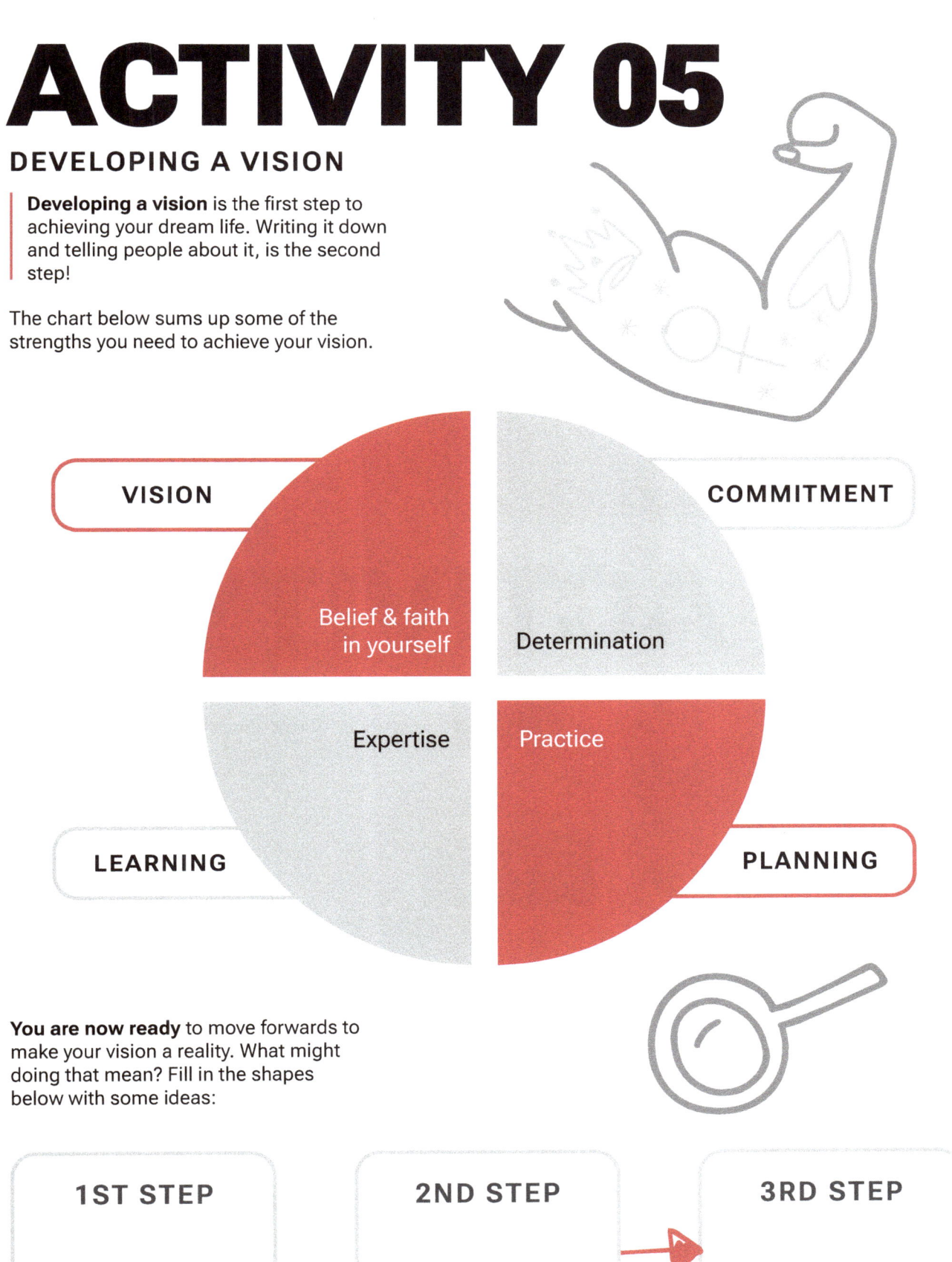

- VISION
- COMMITMENT
- Belief & faith in yourself
- Determination
- Expertise
- Practice
- LEARNING
- PLANNING

You are now ready to move forwards to make your vision a reality. What might doing that mean? Fill in the shapes below with some ideas:

| 1ST STEP | → | 2ND STEP | → | 3RD STEP |

UNIT 08　'YOUR VISION'

ACTIVITY 06

REVIEW YOUR VISION

At home, in your 'Me-Place', go over your work, your vision and your vision statement.

- Does it feel right?
- Do you need to tweak it?
- Can you commit to it?

Once you have your vision statement and are committed to it, you need to keep it alive. **Top tips:**

• Look at it every day to remind yourself of where you are going.

• Share it with your friends and family (otherwise it might disappear)

• Get friends and family to ask you where you are with your plans periodically - this holds us to account!

ACTIVITY 07

eQUALITY CHART

Complete your eQuality chart by inserting your vision into the centre. This could be an image or a text stating 'I am...

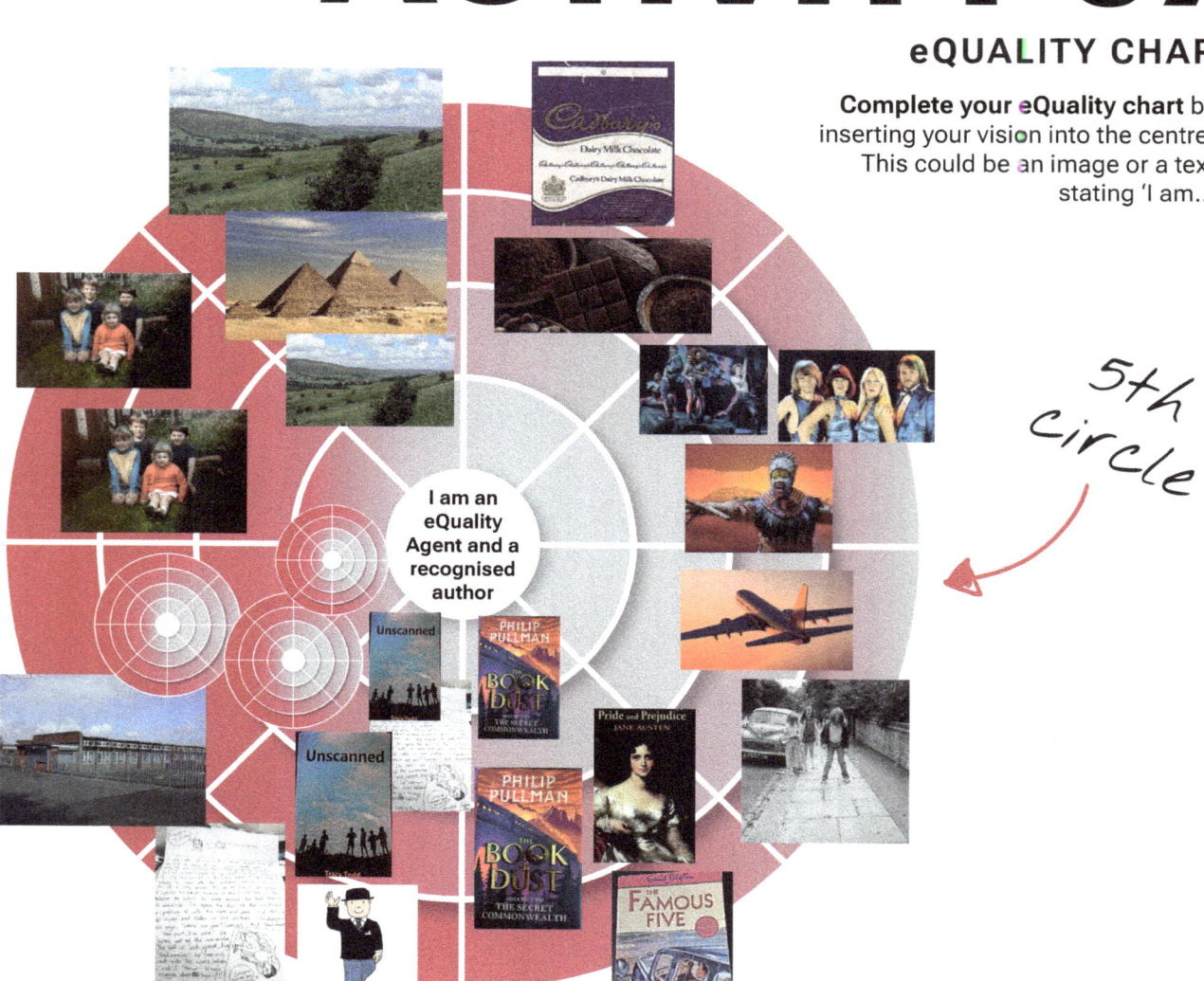

5th circle

74

UNIT 08 'YOUR VISION'

ACTIVITY 08
REVIEW YOUR PROGRESS

Use the boxes below to note what you have learnt so far. Remember, the eQuality Programme is all about you.

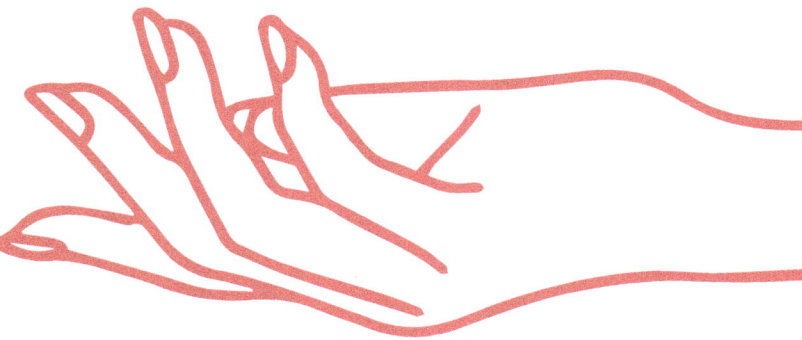

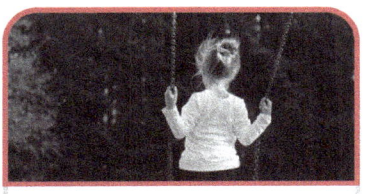

LIKES NOW & THEN

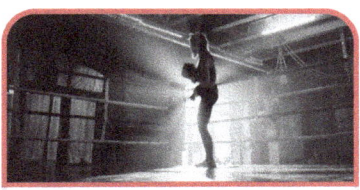

STRENGTHS

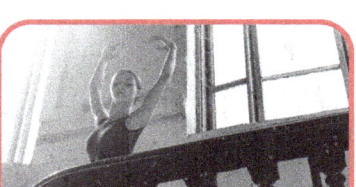

PASSIONS

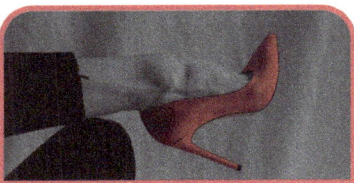

DIG YOUR HEELS IN

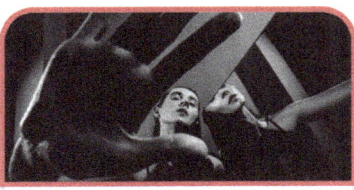

SELF TALK & MINDSET

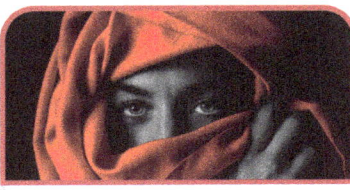

LIFE DREAM & VISION

UNIT 08   'YOUR VISION'

REFLECTIONS
YOUR JOURNEY SO FAR

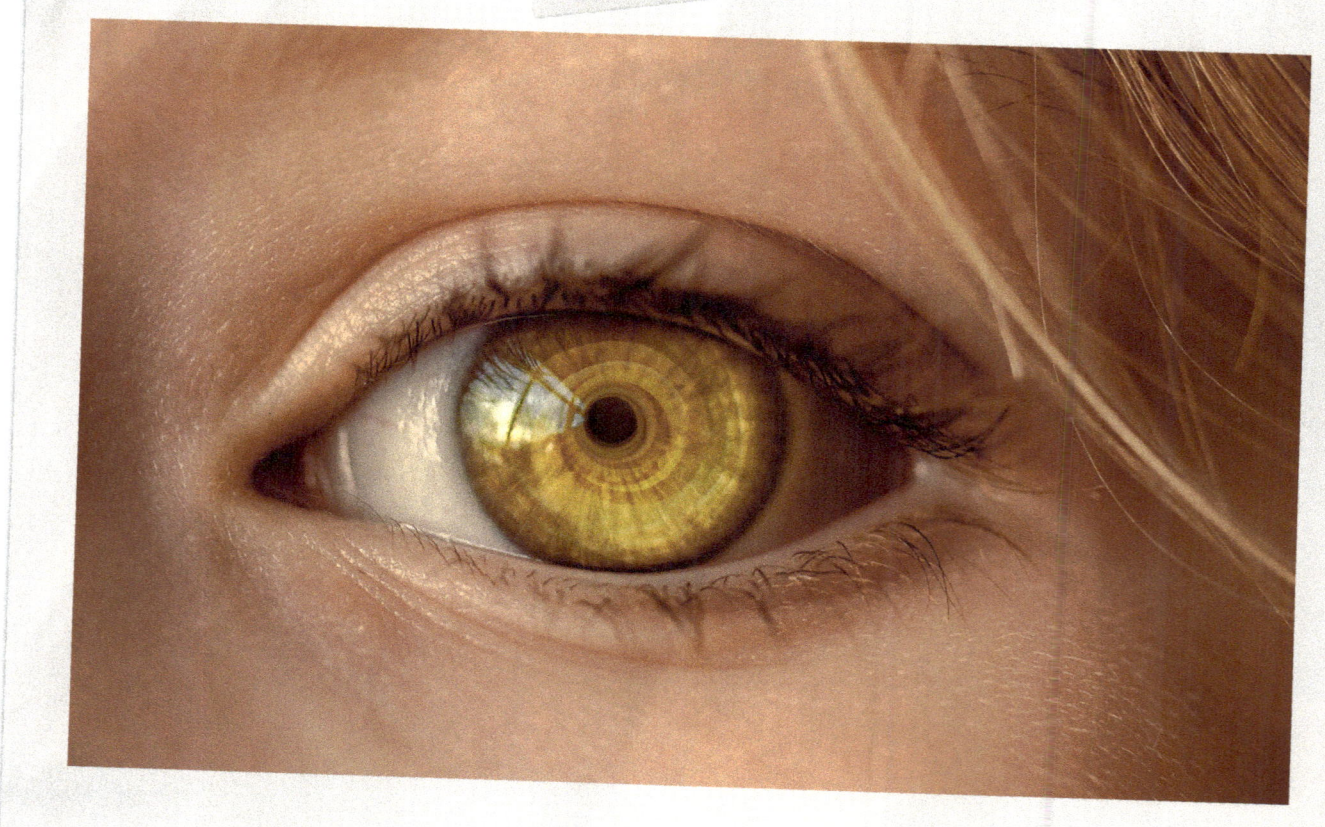

eQUALITY
UNIT #09
'CHUNKING'

The why:
Practicing CHUNKING

We use chunking all the time in so many ways - breaking things down into small steps so we can achieve something bigger. This unit is about exactly that; it's about giving our life vision the same importance as a plan of work.

SOMETIMES THE SMALLEST STEP IN THE RIGHT DIRECTION ENDS UP BEING THE *biggest step* OF YOUR LIFE. TIP TOE IF YOU MUST, BUT *take that step!*

FAIL TO PLAN → PLAN TO FAIL → ~~VISION & DREAMS~~

| UNIT 09   'CHUNKING'

A BEDTIME STORY

There was once a girl whose family was so poor, she received only one bar of chocolate a year on her birthday. (Sound familiar?)

On her twelfth birthday, (January 2nd), she made a decision. Her goal would be to make the bar last the whole year.

How might she do this?

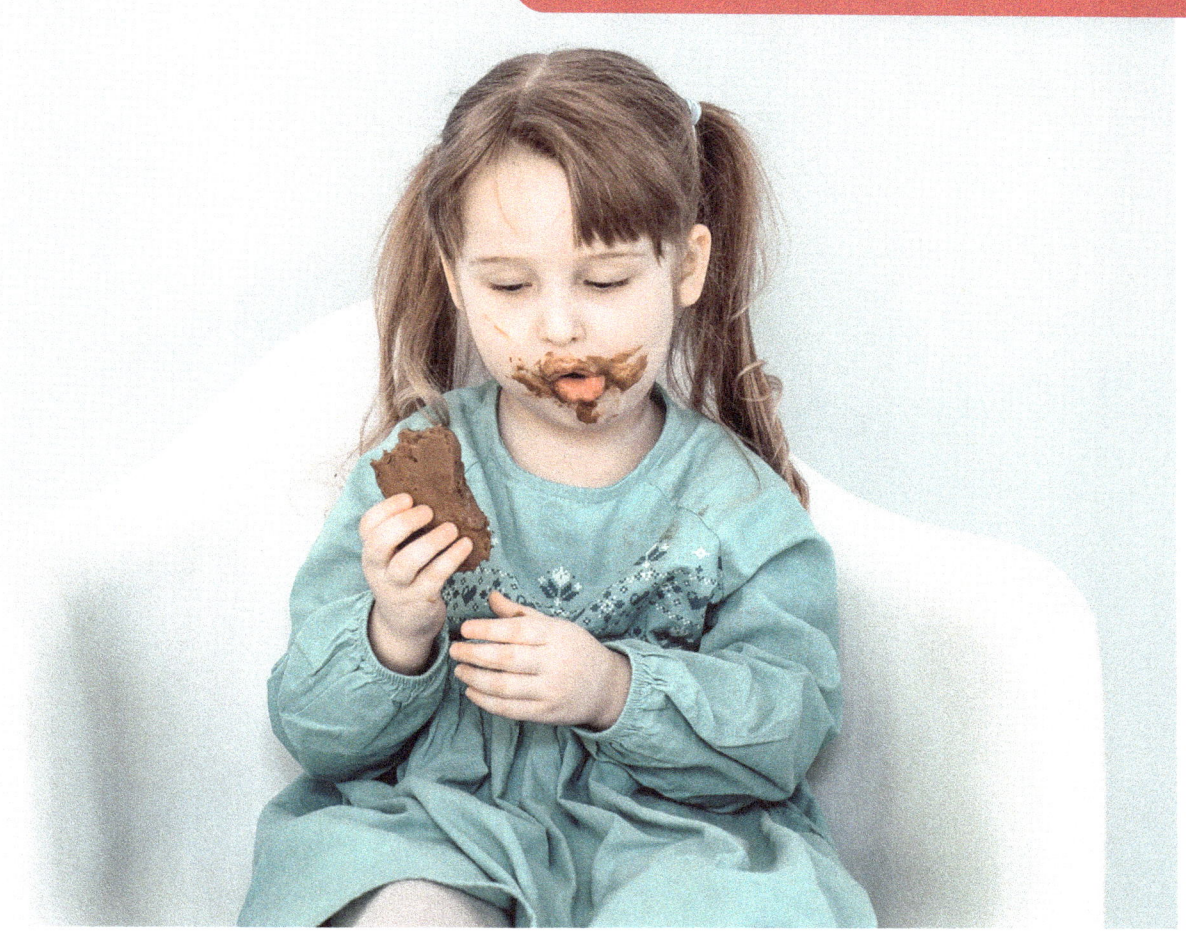

UNIT 09 — 'CHUNKING'

CHUNKING YOUR VISION

Chunking your vision is like eating a chocolate bar one small piece at a time.

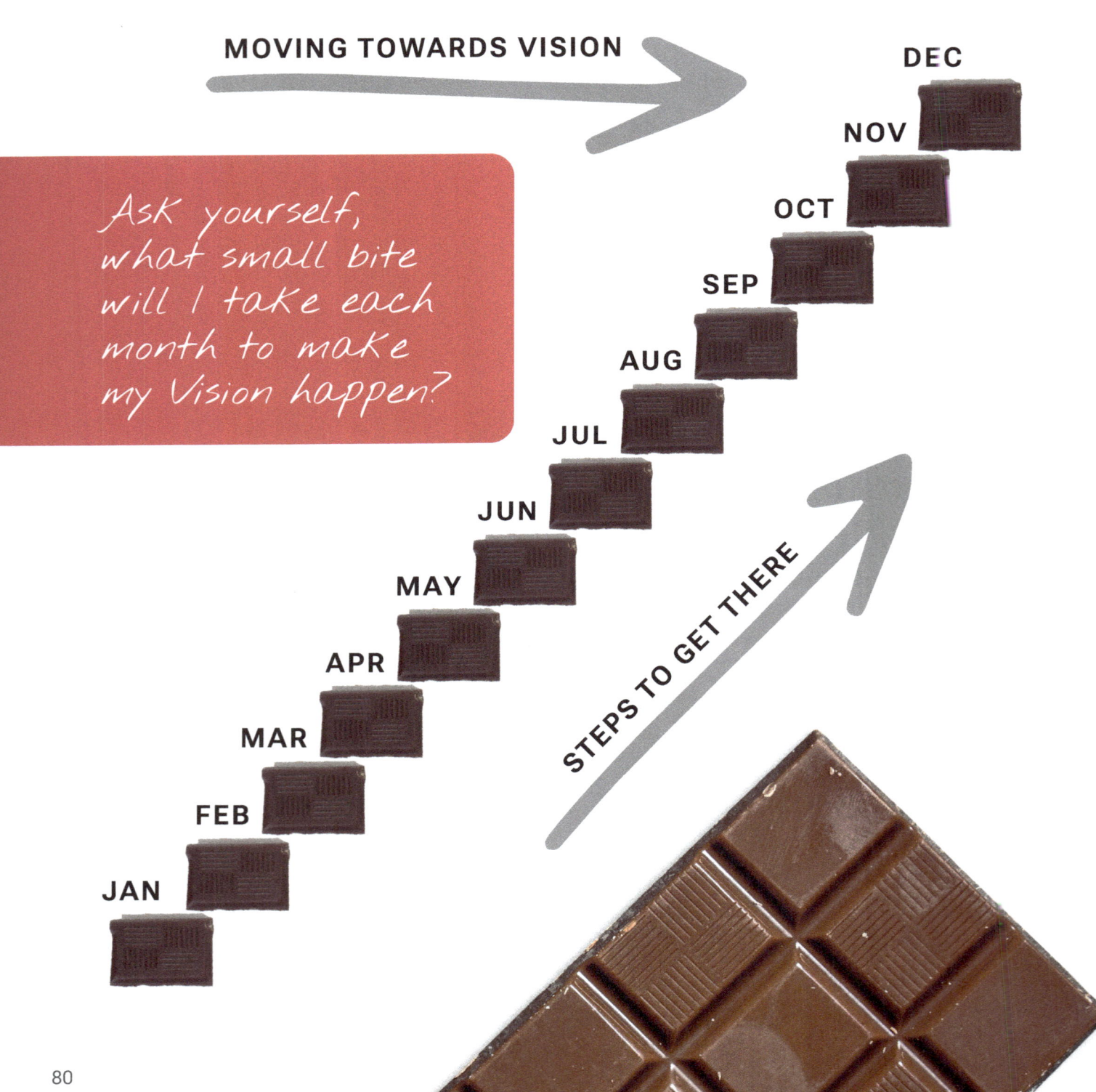

MOVING TOWARDS VISION

Ask yourself, what small bite will I take each month to make my Vision happen?

STEPS TO GET THERE

JAN, FEB, MAR, APR, MAY, JUN, JUL, AUG, SEP, OCT, NOV, DEC

UNIT 09 | 'CHUNKING'

HOW TO CHUNK (1)

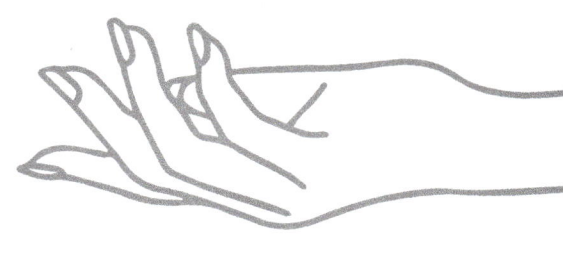

Step 1:

Decide one goal for the first year, (the chocolate bar lasting for a year)

→ This is one of the things that will lead you to achieving your vision. There may be 2 or 3 things in the one year. The vision may take 3 years or more. It's up to you.

EXAMPLE OF STEP 1
Vision: Work in Mental Health Care

GOAL 1
By the end of 20__, I will be in work, or in training/further education which will lead to my preferred job in mental healthcare.

Try to use the 'SMART' method of setting yourself goals and tasks.

What do you think would happen if you set yourself a goal/task you couldn't achieve within the timeframe or one which was not realistic to your current situation?

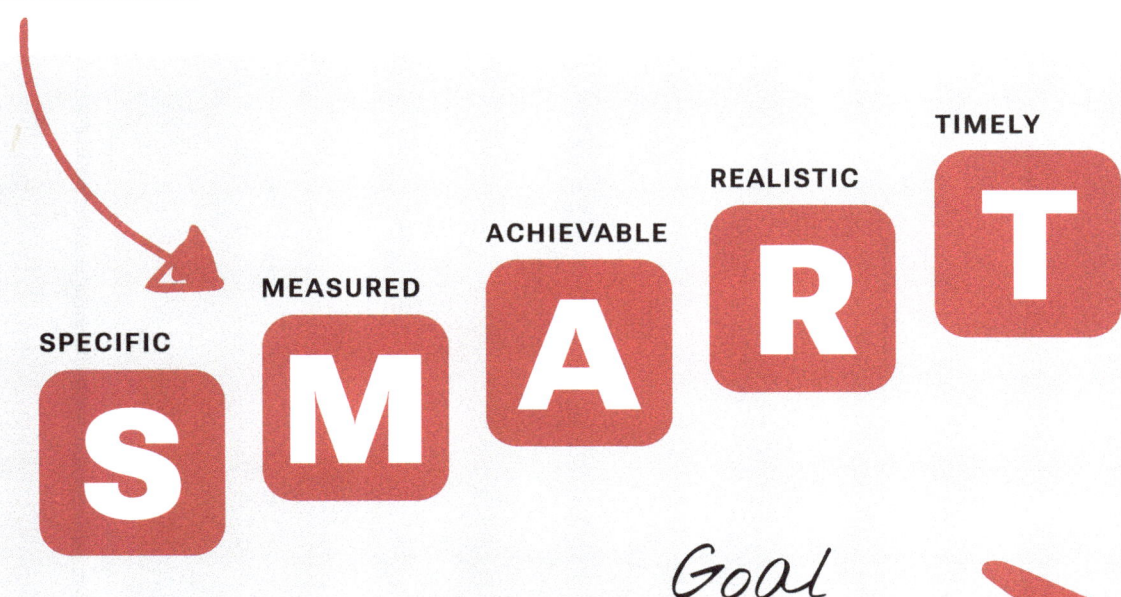

SPECIFIC · MEASURED · ACHIEVABLE · REALISTIC · TIMELY

Goal →

UNIT 09 — 'CHUNKING'

HOW TO CHUNK (2)

Step 2:

Break it down into bite-sized chocolate chunks

Place the chunks in the correct order. What comes first, second etc...

EXAMPLE OF STEP 2
Vision: Work in Mental Health Care

GOAL 1
By the end of 20__, I will be in work, or in training/further education which will lead to my preferred job in mental healthcare.

BITE-SIZED CHUNKS

1. Understand what jobs are in the field and which would interest me by end of November, 20__.

2. Research what training and/or experience I will need by December, 20__ in order to plan ahead.

3. Begin training and/or gain some volunteer work, (or paid if possible), in the area I want to work in by January 20__.

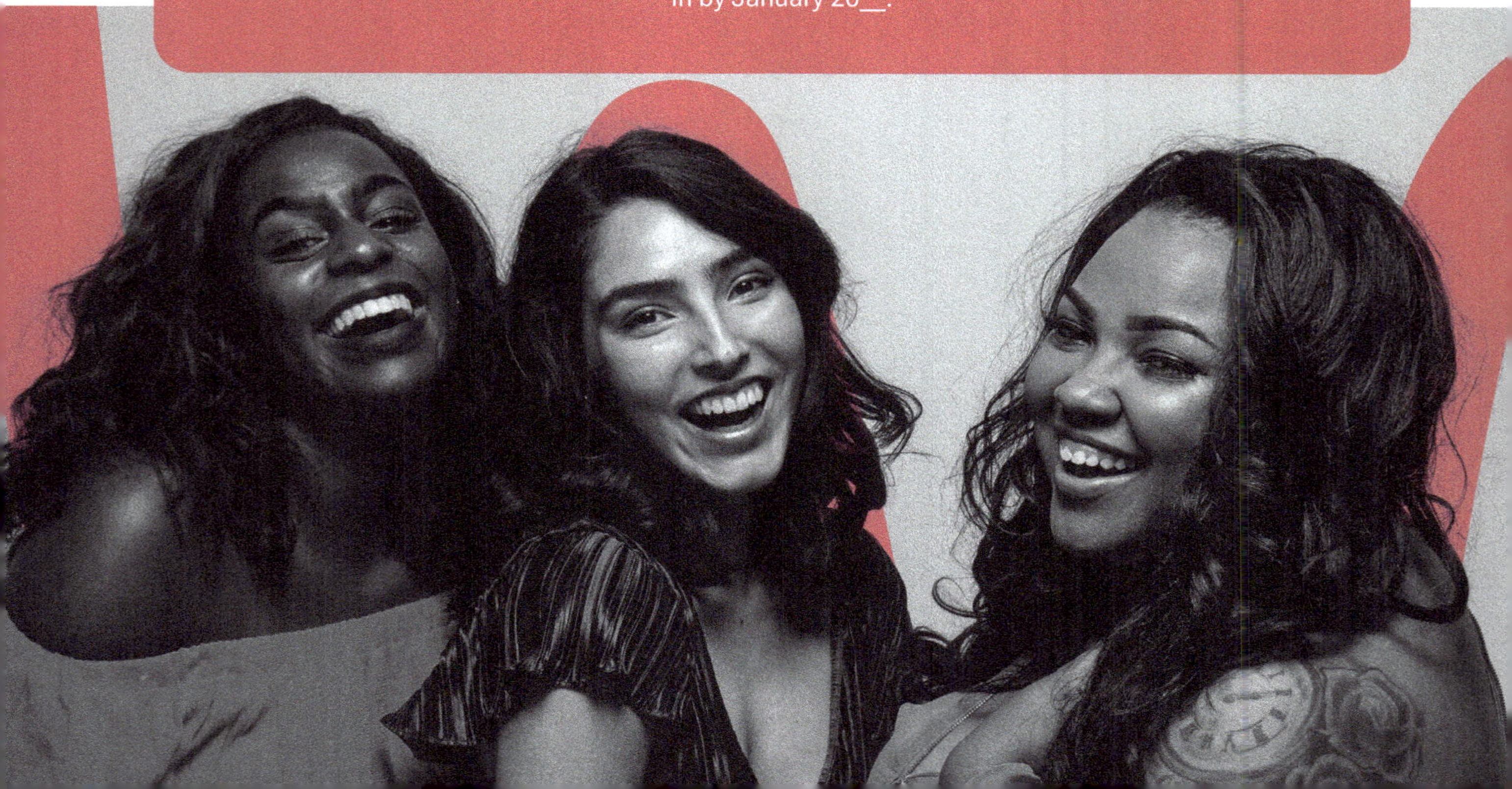

HOW TO CHUNK (3)

Step 3:
Take the bite-sized chocolate chunks and break them down into smaller tasks, (like nibbling at your chocolate bar!).

What you write down at this stage may change when you learn more from research and people you meet. This is okay, but always put a date.

EXAMPLE OF STEP 3
Vision: Work in Mental Health Care

GOAL 1
By the end of 20__, I will be in work, in an apprenticeship or in training/further education which will lead to my preferred job in mental healthcare.

BITE-SIZED CHUNK 1
Understand what jobs are...

Research on line different jobs locally and choose at least three that interest me by 15/11/__.

Call career's advisor by 15/11/__ to make an appointment.

Call local educational Institutes by 15/11/__ to make an appointment.

Research centres that work with those specialities and call them to see if I can have a chat about what is needed by 15/11/__ .

BITE-SIZED CHUNK 2
Research which training...

Have all appointments with careers advisor, education establishments and centres by 31/11/__.

Make a decision about which job I want to do by 5/12/__.

Consider all courses, training apprenticeships, volunteer opportunities and advice given by 5/12/__ and make a decision on the next step.

Decide by 5/12/__ whether to do any volunteer work.

BITE-SIZED CHUNK 3
Begin training...

Begin training, work or volunteering by 15/1/__.

UNIT 09 — 'CHUNKING'

HOW TO CHUNK (4)

Step 4: Review plan

Until you get settled in your job/training/volunteer work, you can review as you learn and change/add more, but don't put things off or put the date too far ahead, or you may lose motivation.

To keep focused, use words in your chunking plan like:

FINISH · COMPLETE · FINALISE · DECIDE

And every time you succeed at one of your tasks, know you have taken a step forwards. Congratulate yourself with little rewards:

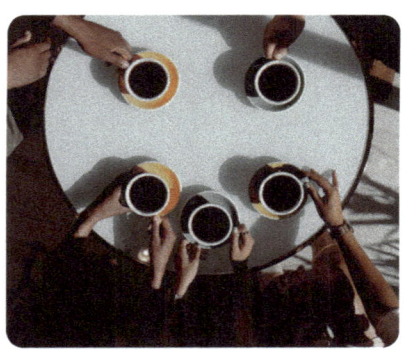
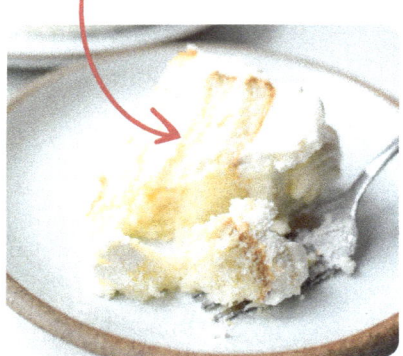
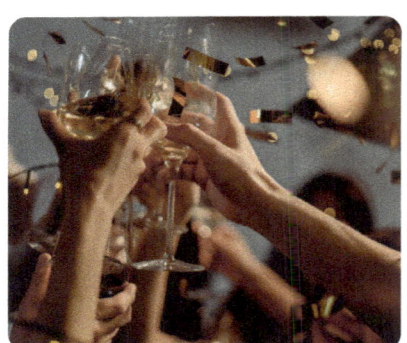
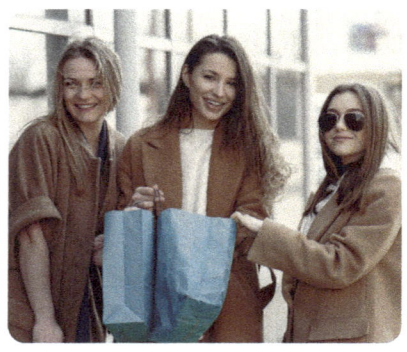
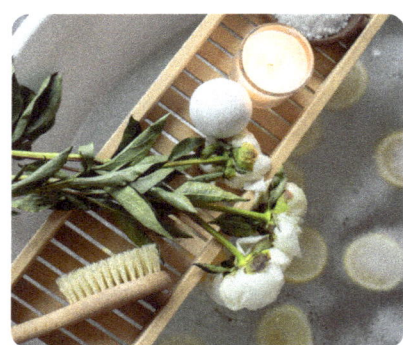
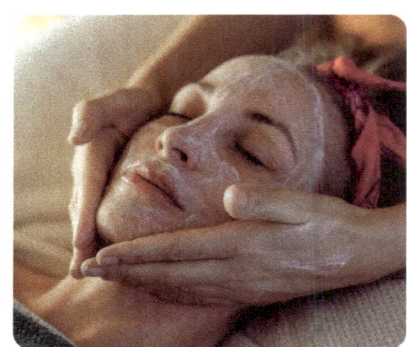

UNIT 09 'CHUNKING'

ACTIVITY 01
COMPLETE THE BELOW

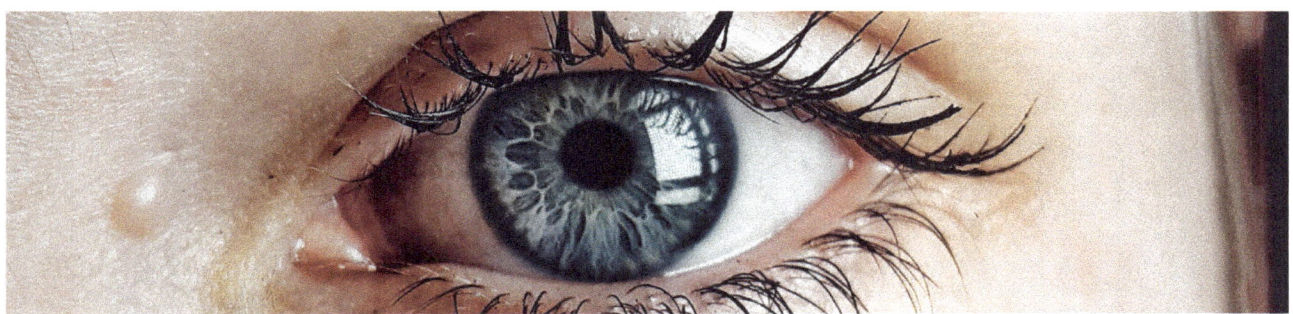

My vision is... _____

_____

STEP 1 - GOAL(S) (End of year)	STEP 2 - BITE-SIZED CHUNKS (In order & dated)
	1.
	2.
	3.
	4.
	5.

| UNIT 09 | | 'CHUNKING' |

STEP 2 - BITE SIZED CHUNKS (Numbers)	STEP 3 - SMALLER TASK WITH FINISHING DATE (Nibbles)	REVIEW
1.		
2.		
3.		
4.		
5.		

UNIT 09 — 'CHUNKING'

ACTIVITY 02
PREPARE A PRESENTATION

Prepare a 5-minute presentation either for yourself or someone else. Stand in front of a mirror if you want, but say it out loud, be proud of what you have achieved.

You could even record it and share with others on the forum/Facebook group page

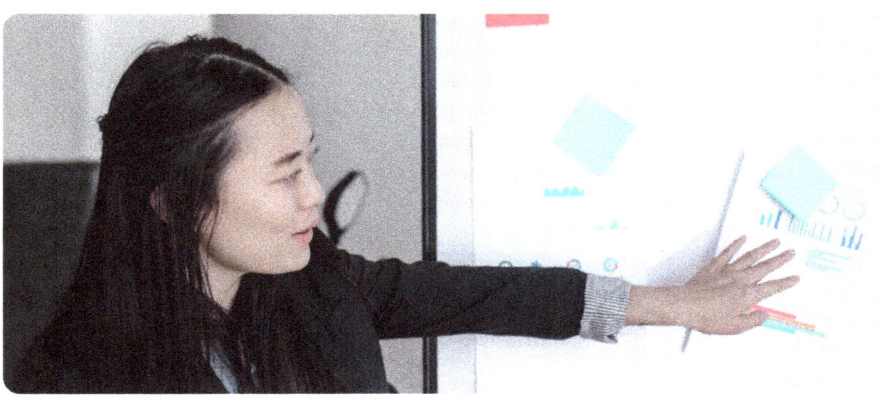

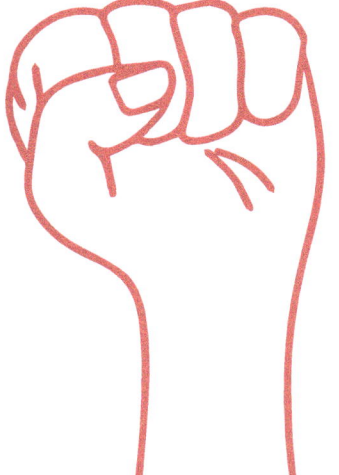

LET'S REVIEW THE WHOLE COURSE

Use your eQuality chart to guide you when thinking about your presentation. Remember all the hard work you have done.

Your eQuality Chart.
a. The links to each circle
b. Your character and ability strengths
c. How you began to understand your passions, dreams and vision

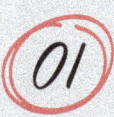

PRESENT YOUR VISION

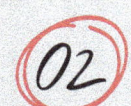

PRESENT YOUR ONE-YEAR GOAL

Present what you have achieved and what you will achieve over the next 3-6 months.

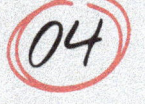

| UNIT 09 | 'CHUNKING' |

REFLECTIONS
YOUR JOURNEY SO FAR

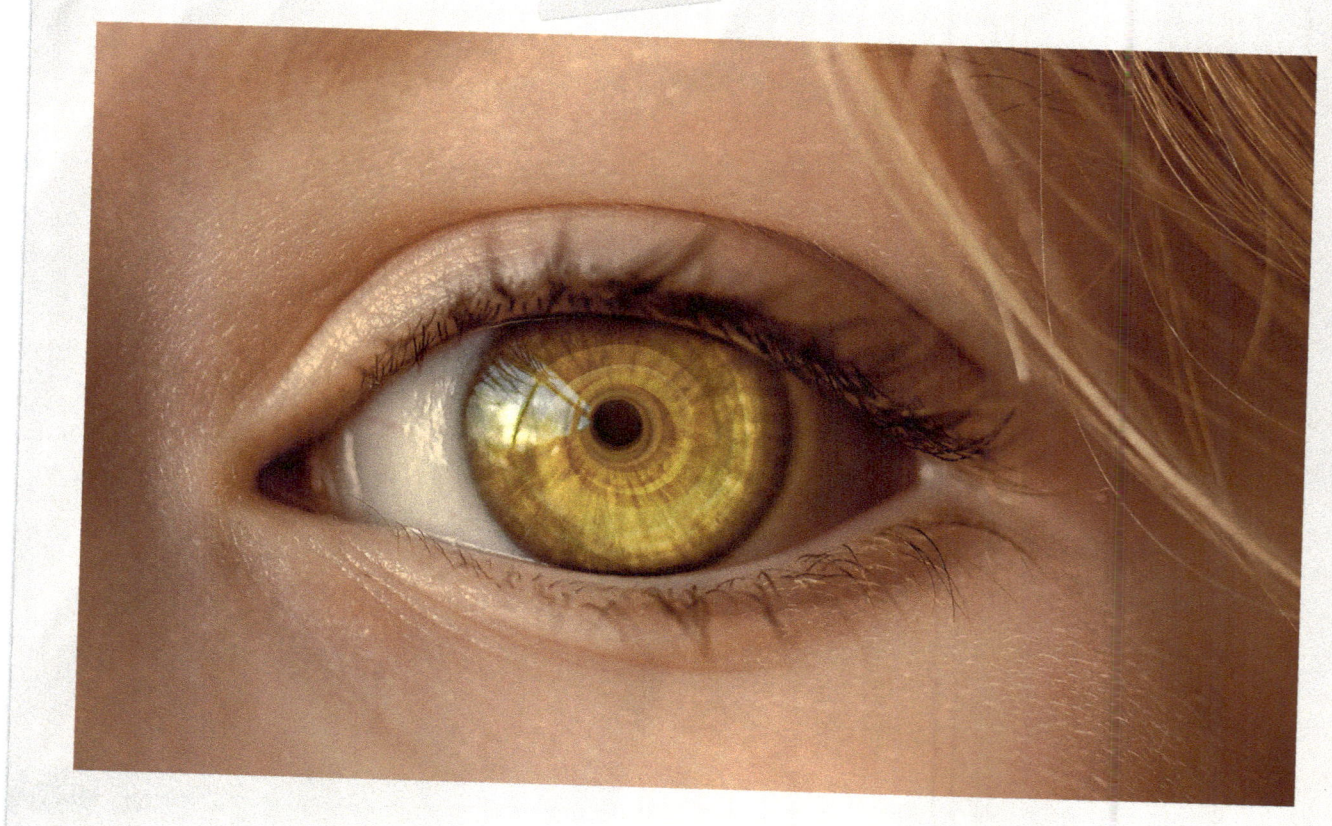

eQUALITY
UNIT #10
'THE FUTURE ME'

The why:
Here's to WHAT'S NEXT

This unit consolidates all your learnings and asks you to consider 'what next?' 'how do I keep moving forwards?' and 'how do I celebrate my successes?' There is also an excellent thought exercise on gratitude and how to benefit mentally from recognising the good things already present in our lives.

UNIT 10 — 'THE FUTURE ME'

ACTIVITY 01
THE CYCLE OF FALLING BACK INTO OLD WAYS OF THINKING

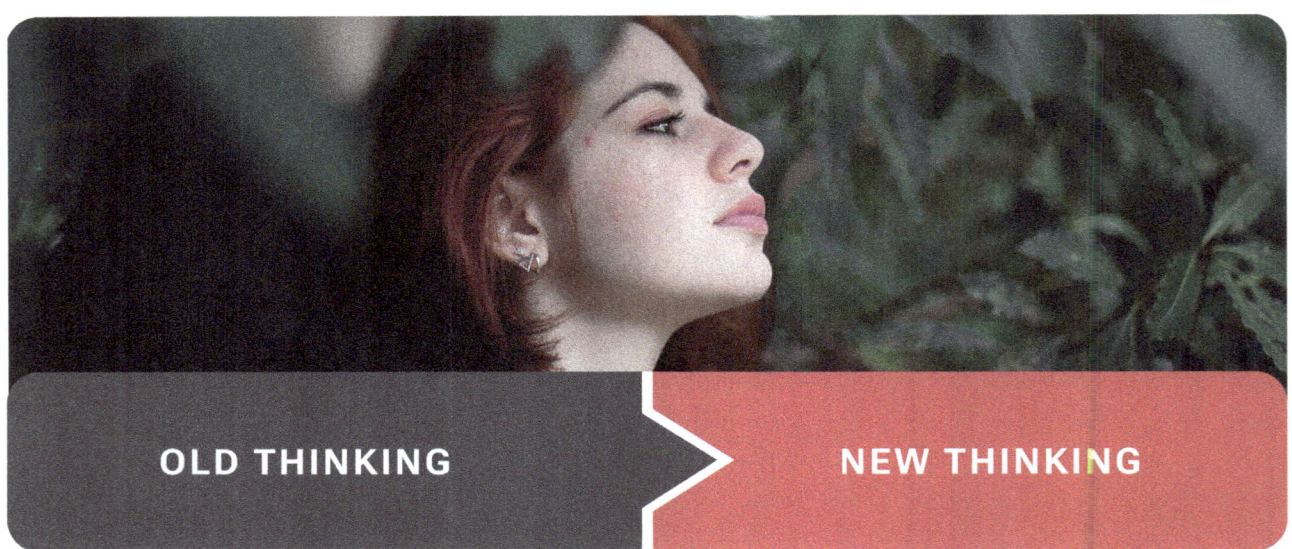

OLD THINKING → NEW THINKING

Recognising the signs

NEW THINKING

OLD THINKING

| UNIT 10 | 'THE FUTURE ME' |

REFLECTION

Reflection is about looking back, evaluating your progress and really understanding how far you've come.

CONSOLIDATION

Consolidation is about bringing it all together, taking those learnings and then moving forward to achieve your dream life.

Don't stop now!

If you stop now, all the work you have done, will be lost. Keep immersing yourself in your new language about what you are, how you see yourself and what steps you are taking to achieve your dreams.

ACTIVITY 02
SUPPORT AND FOLLOW UP

Jot down some ideas in the circles below to think about how you will reflect, consolidate and continue to motivate yourself moving forwards.

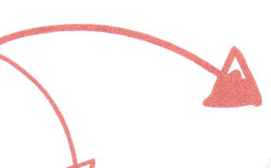

UNIT 10 | 'THE FUTURE ME'

ACTIVITY 03

MOTIVATION - A CLOSER LOOK

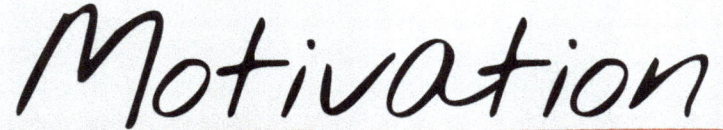
Motivation
The drive to achieve your goals or needs

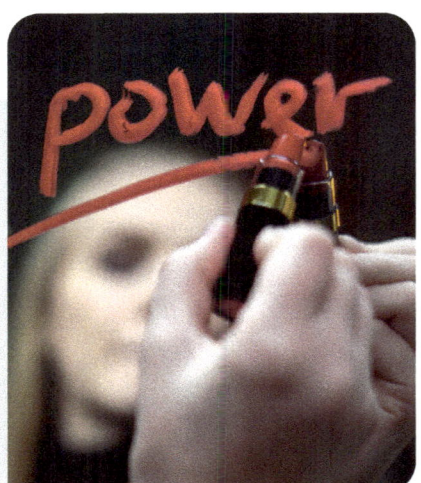

What is it influenced by?
- How much you want the goal
- What you will gain
- What will you lose from not achieving your goal

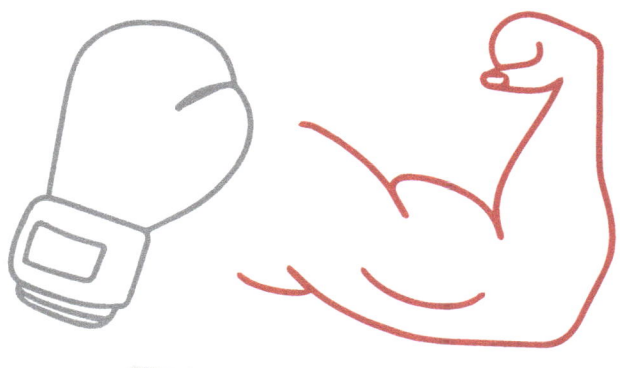

Jot it down, remind yourself.

UNIT 10   'THE FUTURE ME'

SELF-MOTIVATION

FACTORS IN SELF-MOTIVATION

Self-motivation is complex. It's linked to your level of initiative in setting challenging goals for yourself; your belief that you have the skills and abilities needed to achieve those goals; and your expectation that if you put in enough hard work, you will succeed (or at least be in the running, if it's a competitive situation).

Four factors are necessary to build the strongest levels of self motivation:

By working on all of these together, you should quickly improve your self-motivation. Let's look at each of these factors individually.

01 Self-confidence and self-efficacy.

02 Positive thinking about now & positive thinking about the future.

03 Focus and strong goals.

04 A motivating environment.

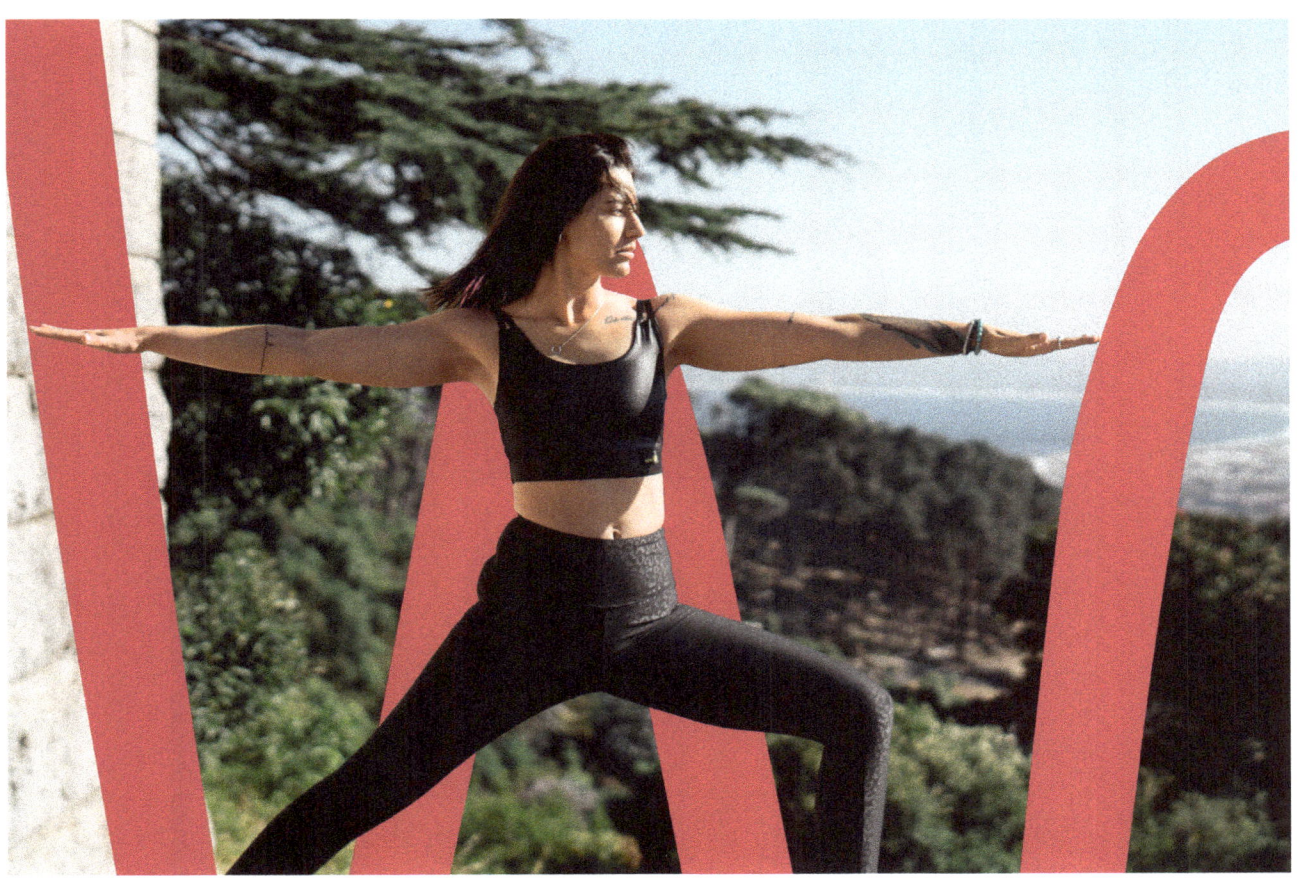

93

01. SELF-CONFIDENCE AND SELF-EFFICACY

> **Albert Bandura**, a psychologist from Stanford University, defined self-efficacy as a belief in our own ability to succeed, and our ability to achieve the goals we set for ourselves. This belief has a huge impact on your approach to goal setting and your behavioural choices as you work toward those goals.

According to Bandura's research, high self-efficacy results in an ability to view difficult goals as a challenge, whereas people with low self-efficacy would likely view the same goals as being beyond their abilities, and might not even attempt to achieve them.

It also contributes to how much effort a person puts into a goal in the first place, and how much he or she perseveres despite setbacks.

By developing a general level of self-confidence in yourself, you will not only believe you can succeed, but you'll also recognise and enjoy the successes you've already had. That, in turn, will inspire you to build on those successes. The momentum created by self-confidence is hard to beat.

Take these steps:

- Think about your achievements in your life.
- Examine your strengths to understand what you can build on.
- Determine what other people see as your strengths and key capabilities.
- Set achievable goals for yourself, work to achieve them, and enjoy both the journey and the achievement.
- Seek out mentors and other people who model the competencies, skills and attributes you desire.

As you begin to recognise how much you've already achieved - and understand how much potential you have - you will have the confidence to set goals and achieve the things you desire. The more you look for reasons to believe in yourself, the easier it will be to find ways to motivate yourself.

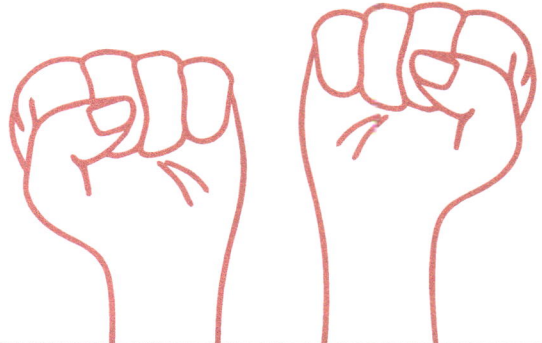

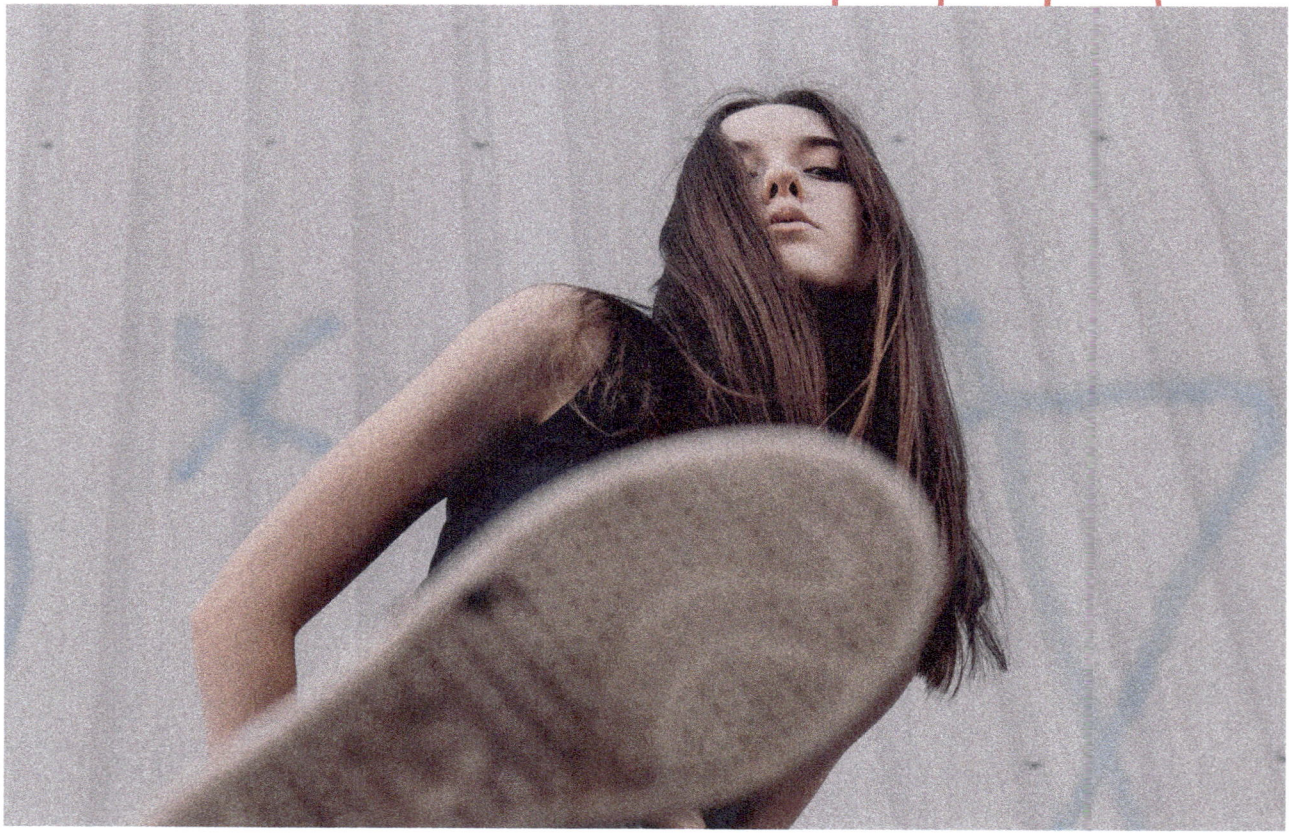

UNIT 10   'THE FUTURE ME'

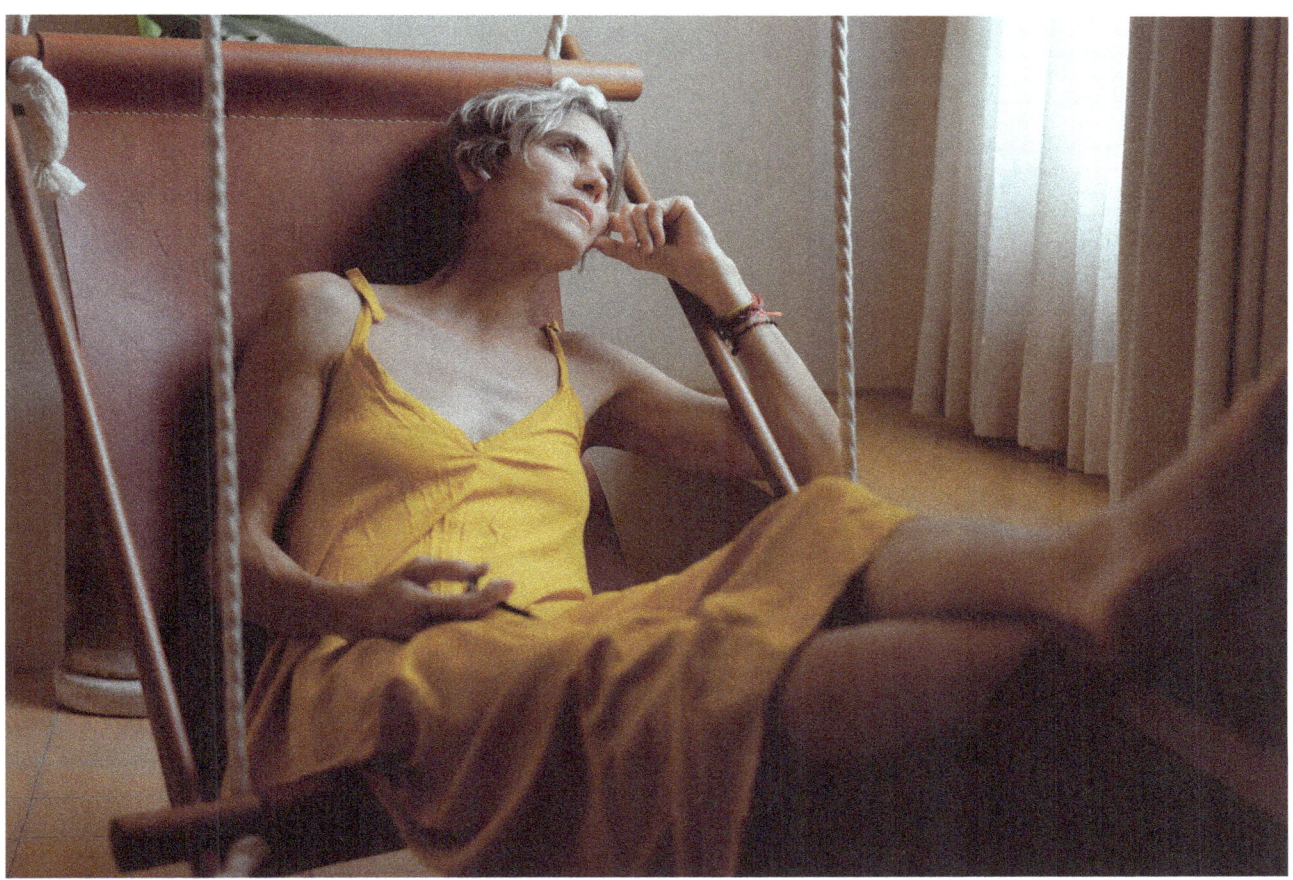

02. POSITIVE THINKING, AND POSITIVE THINKING ABOUT THE FUTURE

> **Your life today is the result of your attitudes and choices in the past.** Your life tomorrow will be the result of your attitudes and the choices you make today.

Positive thinking is closely related to self confidence as a factor in self-motivation. It's important to look at things positively, especially when things aren't going as planned and you're ready to give up.

If you think that things are going to go wrong or that you won't succeed, this may influence outcomes in such a way that your predictions will come true. This is particularly the case if you need to work hard to achieve success, or if you need to persuade others to support you in order to succeed.

Your thoughts can have a major influence on whether you succeed or fail, so make sure those thoughts are 'on your side.' Positive thinking also helps you think about an attractive future that you want to realise.

When you expect positive results, your choices will be more positive, and you'll be less likely to leave outcomes to fate or chance. Having a vivid picture of success, combined with positive thinking, helps you bridge the gap between wanting something and going out to get it.

To apply 'the power of positive thinking', do the following:

- Become aware of your thoughts. Write these down throughout the day.
- Challenge your negative thoughts and replace them with positive ones.
- Create a strong and vivid picture of what it will be like to achieve your goals.
- Develop affirmations or statements that you can repeat to yourself throughout the day. These statements should remind you of what you want to achieve, and why you will achieve it.
- Practice positive thinking until you automatically think about yourself and the world in a positive way, every day.

03. FOCUS AND STRONG GOALS

> **As we've said, a key part of building self-motivation is to start setting strong goals.** These give you focus, a clear sense of direction, and the self-confidence that comes from recognising your own achievement.

First, determine your direction through effective goal setting.

When you set a goal, you make a promise to yourself. Part of the strength of this is that it gives you a clear direction. Also, once you've made this promise to yourself, you'll want to keep it. And that is the challenge. Remember, the journey is as important as meeting the challenge. Have fun along the way!

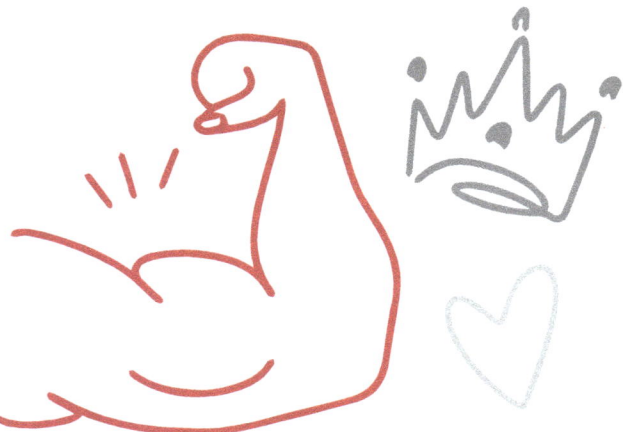

Don't set just any goal. According to Locke's goal-setting theory, your goal should have the following characteristics:

- **Clarity** - Effective goals are clear, measurable, specific, and based on behaviour, not outcomes.
- **Challenge** - Goals should be difficult enough to be interesting, but not so difficult that you can't reach them.
- **Commitment** - Goals should be attainable, and should be relevant - that is, they should contribute in a significant way to the major objectives you're trying to achieve.
- **Regularity of Feedback** - Monitor your progress towards your goals regularly to maintain your sense of momentum and enthusiasm, and enjoy your progress towards those goals.
- **Sufficient Respect for Complexity** - If the goal involves complex work, make sure that you don't over-commit yourself. Complex work can take an unpredictably long time to complete (particularly if you have to learn how to do the task 'on the job').

When you have a variety of goals, be sure to schedule your time and resources effectively. You can achieve the 'focus' part of self-motivation by prioritising and establishing a schedule that will help you succeed. It doesn't make sense to work until you're exhausted or give up one goal to achieve another.

04. MOTIVATING ENVIRONMENT

> **The final thing to focus on** is surrounding yourself with people and resources that will remind you of your goals, and help you with your internal motivation.

These are external factors - they'll help you get motivated from the outside, which is different from the internal motivation discussed so far. However, the more factors you have working for you, the better.

You can't just rely on these 'environmental' or outside elements alone to motivate you, but you can use them for extra support.

Try the following:

- Look for teamwork opportunities. Working in a team makes you accountable to others.
- Ask your boss for specific targets and objectives to help you measure your success.
- Ask for interesting assignments.
- Set up some goals that you can easily achieve. Quick wins are great for getting you motivated.
- Buddy up with people who you trust to be supportive, and ask them to help keep you accountable.
- Try not to work by yourself too much. Balance the amount of time you work from home with time spent working with others.

UNIT 10 — 'THE FUTURE ME'

KEY POINTS
SELF-MOTIVATION

Self-motivation doesn't come naturally to everyone. And even those who are highly self-motivated need some extra help every now and then.

Build your self-motivation by practising goal-setting skills, and combining those with positive thinking, the creation of powerful visions of success, and the building of high levels of self-efficacy and self-confidence.

Your attitude and beliefs about your likelihood of success can predict whether or not you actually succeed.

Set goals, and work hard to achieve them. Examine ways to improve your self-motivation, and regularly reassess your motivation levels.

If you actively keep your internal motivation high, you can significantly increase the likelihood of achieving your hopes, dreams, and visions of the future.

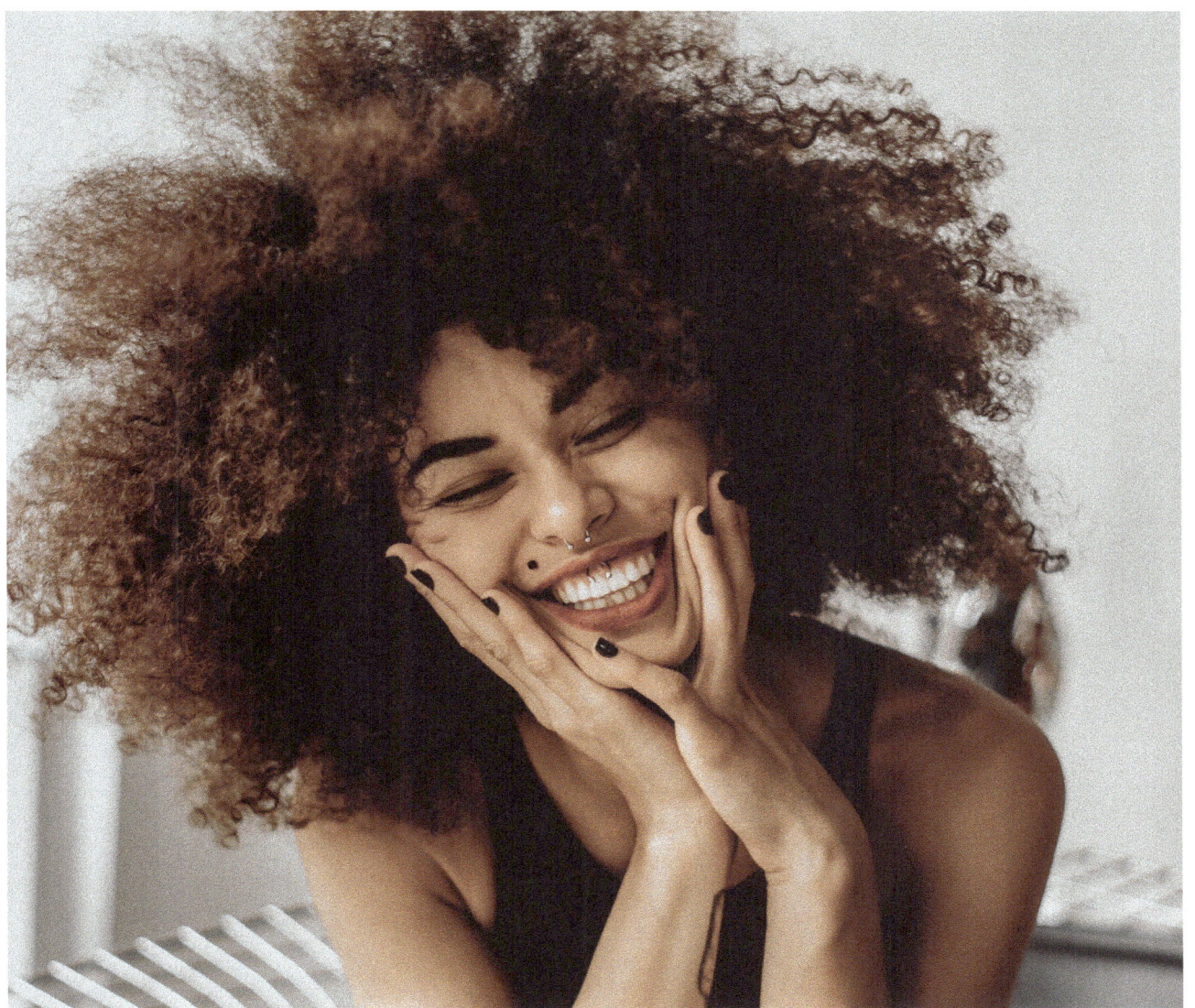

| UNIT 10 'THE FUTURE ME' |

ACTIVITY 04
IF YOU LOSE MOTIVATION

I'll not beat myself up, it's normal. I'll list my achievements. I'll remember how I've failed and achieved over and over. Resilience helps. We can carry on and continue from where I left off.

Things I will do:

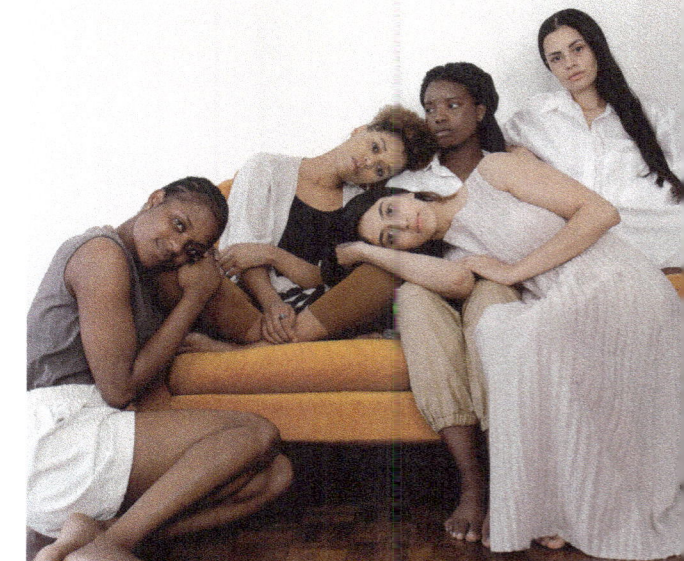

Review goals and see if they are realistic in the timeframe set. You may need to break your goal down further into smaller and more achievable goals.

Remember why you wanted to get motivated or reach that goal in the first place.

Seek motivation from others – read a motivational book. Talk to a friend, family or even a mentor who has reached similar goals to the ones you have set.

Sometimes taking a break and starting afresh is also what is needed.

FINDING MOTIVATION WHEN WE LOSE IT

UNIT 10　　　　　　　　　　　　　　　　　　　　　　　　'THE FUTURE ME'

ACTIVITY 05
GRATITUDE JOURNAL

Keeping a journal of gratifying experiences is a key to living a more full-filled life. There's no wrong way to complete a Gratitude Journal. But here are a couple of pointers to help you get started.

Use the Gratitude Journal to record 5 things you are grateful for each day.

Identify 1 extra item each day that you've never expressed gratitude for before. Keep this journal handy and reference at a moment of low self-esteem, or when you are struggling to feel thankful.

Read through previous entries and take note of any emotional shifts.

DATE		TODAY, I AM GRATEFUL FOR...	SOMETHING I NEED TO EXPRESS GRATITUDE FOR...
	1.		
	2.		
	3.		
	4.		
	5.		
	1.		
	2.		
	3.		
	4.		
	5.		
	1.		
	2.		
	3.		
	4.		
	5.		

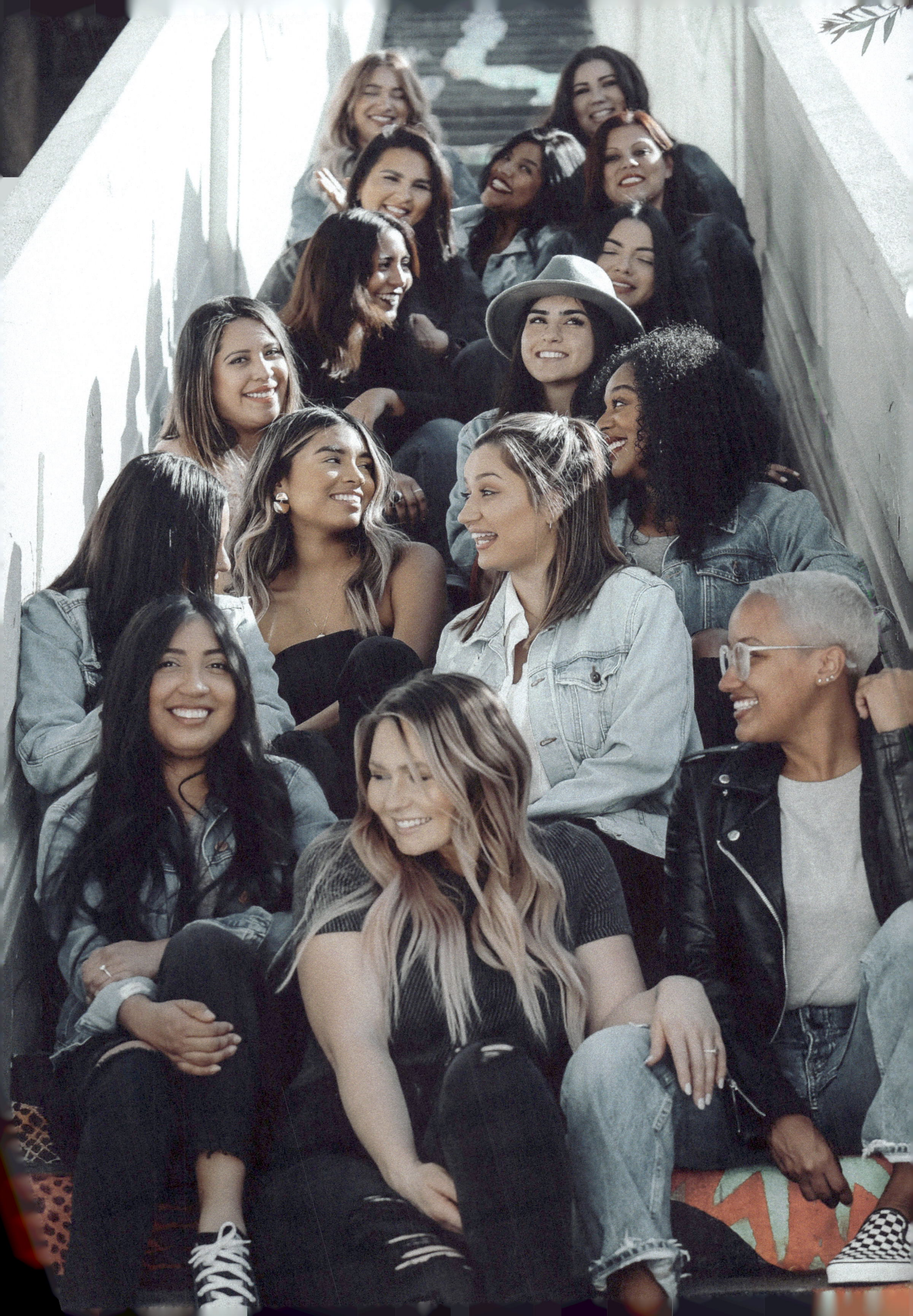

eQUALITY
THANK YOU

We would like to thank you for choosing the eQuality Personal Development Programme.

As with all good journeys, this one must end, and you must continue with your journey towards your version of success.

It has been our pleasure to be part of your development. We wish you well and look forward to working with you in the future, and of course hearing all about your success.

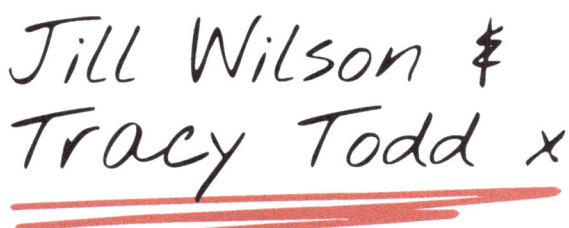

Jill Wilson & Tracy Todd x

www.ingramcontent.com/pod-product-compliance
Lightning Source LLC
Chambersburg PA
CBHW042015090526
44587CB00028B/4271